Intermittent Fasting for Women Over 50

The Only Weight Loss Guide that Actually Helps Women Reset their Metabolism, Burn Fat, Balance Hormones and Live Longer - Follow the 16/8 Method for a Complete Body Detox!

By

Nancy Johnson

work can be in any fashion deemed liable for any hardship or damages that may befall them after undertaking information described herein.

Additionally, the information in the following pages is intended only for informational purposes and should thus be thought of as universal. As befitting its nature, it is presented without assurance regarding its prolonged validity or interim quality. Trademarks that are mentioned are done without written consent and can in no way be considered an endorsement from the trademark holder.

Table of Contents

Introduction

Most women over 50 feel as if they have lost their ability to be attractive, healthy and feel good in their own bodies. But what is the cause for this widespread issue? The fact is that in today's world we are spending more and more time at home and we have significantly reduced our need for food. However, even if we do not need as many calories as we did in the past to survive and be healthy, most of us are still eating as if they were running a marathon a day.

Therefore, it should not come as a surprise that most women over 50 years of age are out of shape, overweight and unhealthy. This normally translates into a worse quality of life and is something that is frustrating for a substantial portion of the female population. Thanks to researches and scientific studies conducted by incredible nutritionists, it is now possible to overcome the negative effect of a sedentary life. In fact, intermittent fasting seems like the perfect solution for all those women that want to burn fat, lose weight and gain a healthy and new lifestyle.

The need of all these women is what inspired the writing of this guide. In fact, in the next chapters you are not going to find complicated explanations of scientific topics that, even if interesting, do not give you a clear direction on what you can do to start feeling better. On the contrary, while writing this book, a great effort was made to make sure that each concept is followed by a subsequent strategy that can be implemented in a healthy intermittent fasting protocol.

By reading this book you will get all the information and practical steps you need to follow to start intermittent fasting in just a few days. We advise you to talk to your doctor before changing your diet as intermittent fasting is not suitable if you have certain healthy conditions.

Please, be aware that the goal of this book is to give you accurate information on intermittent fasting, but it does not take the place of a true medical advice. We hope that you can find motivational and informative insights that help you make a change for the better.

To your success!

Nancy Johnson

Chapter 1 - The most Important Component: Mindset

One of the most important tools at your disposal when you decide to lose weight and win a healthier lifestyle is your ability to make long lasting changes to your routine. In order to do this, you need to have a positive and effective mindset that can sustain you when things get difficult. That is why we have decided to dedicate the first few chapters of this book to this extremely important topic.

The willpower, also known as self-discipline, self-control or determination, is the ability to control your behaviors, emotions and focus. The willpower involves the ability to resist impulses and sacrifice immediate gratification in order to achieve your goals. It also includes the ability to ignore unwelcome thoughts, feelings or impulses, as well as that of self-regulation. The level of willingness of a woman can determine its ability to save for its financial stability, to make positive choices for its mental and physical health and to avoid the use or abuse of harmful substances. Continuing to give up instant gratifications in favor of future prizes, you can move towards your goals and develop your willpower. Thanks to a constant "workout" of the mind, this practice will strengthen your ability to control your impulses, exactly how physical exercise strengthens your muscles.

Let's take a look at some tips that can help you build up your mindset.

Evaluate your habits

If you are trying to improve your willpower, probably your inability to control your impulses is negatively affecting some areas of your life. Some women over 50 struggle with their willpower in every aspect of their life, while others are limited to having some specific "weaknesses". Determine what the area you intend to improve and, if the areas are a lot, choose to dedicate yourself to one at a time.

For example, your willpower could be weak in front of the food. This could consequently negatively affect your health and quality of your life For example, you may have difficulty following your intermittent fasting protocol, which causes you to binge and not be healthy. Whatever health issue you are facing today, acknowledging it is the first step to overcome it.

Create a scale to evaluate your willpower

You will need to evaluate your willpower as efficiently as possible during your intermittent fasting protocol. You could create a scale from 1 to 10, in which 1 represents a complete indulgence relative to the thing, or to things, that you are trying to avoid, and 10 a stoic respect for the restrictive rules that you have established for yourself. Alternatively you can develop a simpler scale, based on "at all, little, more, much". This scale can take different forms, while continuing to offer you the opportunity to evaluate yourself while following an intermittent fasting protocol.

For example, if you realize you eat sweets in a compulsive way or stop in some fast food restaurants on a daily basis, on a scale from 1 to 10 you can evaluate yourself with a 1 or a 2.

Think long term

If you want to improve yourself, the first step to take is to set a goal for your change. You will need to choose a clear, specific and achievable goal. If it were too vague or not measurable, it would indeed be difficult to determine any progress made or establish it achieved.

For example, the "eating healthier" goal, established by those women who tend to eat impulsively, will certainly be too vague. "Healthier" is a relative concept, which will make it difficult to establish when it was reached. A more concrete destination could be to "lose 20 pounds through a healthy intermittent fasting protocol", "return to a size 44" or "overcoming my sugar addiction ".

Have short term goals as well

When you want to reach an important goal (which could appear complicated), one of the best ways to do this is to establish intermediate goals along the way. Your short-term goals must also be specific and measurable, and able to lead you to your final goal.

For example, if you are trying to lose 20 pounds, you can give you a first short-term goal similar to "losing 5 pounds", "do exercise 3 times a week" or "limit desserts to once a week".

Think big

The best way to "train" your willpower is to show you are willing to sacrifice the desire for immediate gratification in favor of a better long-term reward. The final compensation will be that of "living well" or "feeling attractive"; However, to learn how to exercise your willpower it is advisable to establish a concrete prize.

For example, if your desire is to lose weight, trying to control your compulsive hunger through a healthy intermittent fasting protocol, your final reward could be a new dress that makes you feel amazing.

Give up immediate gratification

This is the essence of the development of willpower. When you feel tempted to give up to an impulse, realize that what you really want to live is that short feeling of immediate gratification. In case your impulsive behavior is contrary to your goals, after giving away to immediate gratification you will feel guilty.

To resist the desire for immediate gratification, follow these steps.

- Recognize what you want to do.
- Admit that the only thing you want is immediate gratification.
- Remember your short and long-term goals you set for yourself.
- Ask yourself if it's worth giving to the current impetus and jeopardize your journey towards the ultimate goal.

For example, if you are working to keep nervous hunger under control by following a healthy intermittent fasting protocol and during a party you find yourself in front of a tray full of biscuits, do the following things.

- Feel how much you would like to eat those biscuits.
- Recognize that that biscuit could be able to satisfy your current desire for sweets.
- Remember yourself that you are working to achieve the goal of losing 20 pounds by following intermittent fasting protocol and the reward of a new wardrobe.
- Ask yourself if temporary satisfaction given by that biscuit deserves to renounce the progress made and the potential loss of the final award.

Give yourself small rewards for the results achieved

A motivation or reward system will not change your long-term will strength, but you can help you follow the way to success. Since the achievement of a final goal may take a long time, it could be effective to set small rewards for the progress made so that they act as motivation to keep going.

For example, if for a week you have followed your intermittent fasting protocol, you can give yourself a small dose of your favorite dessert over the weekend. Alternatively, you can reward you with something that is not bound to food, like a pedicure or a massage.

Notes your attempts to check your impulses, including both the successful ones and the unsuccessful ones. Don't forget those details that in the future could help you evaluate the situation.

For example, you could write: "Today I ate five cookies during an office party. I had missed lunch and I was quite hungry. I was surrounded by many people and Sara, who had prepared the cookies, repeatedly encouraged me to eat one of them".

Comment on the factors that influenced your decision-making process

In addition to detailing the situation you have resisted or how you have surrendered to the impulse, describe what has passed through your mind in those moments. You may want to include your emotional state, the people you were next to you and the place where you were there.

After describing several episodes in your diary, you can start to re-read them, trying to highlight possible schemes in your behaviors. Here are some questions you should ask yourself.

- Is my decision-making process more effective when I am alone or when I am with other people?
- Are there some people who more than others "trigger" my compulsive behaviors?
- Do my emotions (depression, anger, happiness, etc.) influence my compulsive behavior?
- Is there a particular moment of the day when it is more difficult to keep my impulses under control?

You can decide to create a visual representation of your progress

It may seem to be a strange idea, but there are many women who respond better to a more concrete visual representation of their progress. It will be easier to remain motivated by having something that clearly shows you the many steps taken so far, as well as those still to be done.

For example, if you want to lose 20 pounds, you can insert a coin in a jar whenever you lose 0,5 lbs. Seeing the level of coins grow while losing weight you will have a concrete representation of the progress made.

Find out what is more effective for you

By reading your diary or simply reflecting on your successes and your false steps, you can realize what is more useful for you. You may notice that giving you a weekly reward is really effective. You could then find that being alone is a triggering cause of your compulsive behavior, or that you find yourself in a given place or in the presence of certain people contribute to increasing your food cravings. Customize your approach to increase your willpower based on your specific needs.

Stress can hinder your progress

Whatever health your goal you are trying to reach, stress deriving from working or personal life has the potential to derail your progress. Therefore, it could be necessary to use techniques to reduce your stress. Do not underestimate the influence stress can have in your ability to follow your intermittent fasting protocol.

Sometimes the best way to defeat temptation is to avoid it. If you feel you don't have the willpower needed to resist your compulsive behavior, try to eliminate the opportunity to give up your intermittent fasting protocol. This could mean wanting to avoid those people or those environments that tend to trigger your cravings. This solution may not be valid long-term, but prove to be useful in the beginning of your intermittent fasting protocol or during some particularly difficult moments.

For example, if you tend to eat outside your scheduled eating window, you can decide to empty your home of all sorts of unhealthy food. Remove from your pantry everything that does not suit your new healthy habits, throwing it away.

Use "if-then" affirmations

You can "mentally feel" your reactions at a given situation by inventing some scenarios in advance using the "if-then" structure. Doing this will be particularly useful when you will find yourself in a situation that tempts you.

For example, if you are about to attend a party where biscuits will be available, you can use the following "if - then" statement. "If Sara will offer me a biscuit, then I gently tell her 'no, thanks, but they look delicious' and I'll move to the other side of the room".

Search for medical help

If you have been trying without success to keep your impulses at bay, evaluate the hypothesis to turn to a therapist. They can offer you support and specific tips to change your behaviors.

People suffering from obsessive or compulsive behavior or dependencies can benefit from the help of a therapist specialized in impulse control disorders or cognitive pathologies.Some impulse control disorders and some deficiencies in the willpower can also benefit from a treatment known as "Habit Reversal Therapy" which replaces unwanted habit with another more useful habit.

Chapter 2 - How to Set Your Goals

Whether you have small dreams or high expectations from your intermittent fasting protocol, having goals will allow you to plan your path through this weight loss journey. The achievement of some goals can require a whole life, while others can be conquered from morning to evening. Whatever your goals, broad and generic or specific and practical, in reaching them you will feel satisfied and you will see your self-esteem grow. If the fulfillment of the first necessary steps intimidates you, continue reading and find out how to consolidate the widest desire.

Determine the goals for your life

Ask yourself important questions regarding what you want to get from life. On a physical level, you might want to be back in shape by following an intermittent fasting protocol.

Analyze the areas in which, over time, you would like to make changes or improvements. Start wondering what you want to get in every specific area, and think about what steps you want to take in the next five years.

In the case of the goal "I want to get back in shape", you could establish minor goals as "I want to follow my intermittent fasting protocol" and "I want to fast at least 16 hours a day".

Once you know what you want to get over the next few years, you have to start taking the steps necessary to reach them by writing down the actual goals.

If you want to get back in shape, your first goal may be to eat more fruits and vegetables and run for 3 miles. We will have a chapter dedicated to writing down your goals in the best possible way, for now just know that it is fundamental if you want to lose weight and keep it off.

You have to highlight the reasons why you have decided to set such a goal and reflect on what will happen once you reach it. For example, if referring to a short-term fitness goal you have decided to achieve, it is good to ask yourself if and how your choice will help you reach your main health goal. If necessary, evaluate to change your short-term goal by replacing it with a practice that allows you to effectively advance towards the final destination.

Periodically check your goals

Instead of limiting you to remain anchored on your initial positions, from time to time find time to re-evaluate your minor goals. Are you respecting the temporal deadlines you have set for yourself? Are the steps planned able to lead you to your finish line? Be flexible in changing and adapting your minor goals.

To get back in shape, you may have to follow an intermittent fasting protocol for several weeks. If you start by following a 16/8 intermittent fasting protocol it might be the case for you to take things to a new level by committing yourself to an 18/6 protocol. Have fixed goals but do not be afraid to change your approach to reach them faster.

Make your goals specific

When you set a goal, you have to make sure that you respond to very specific questions: who, what, where and why. For any goal you set, you should reflect on your reasons and ask you how it helps to get you to achieve what you want in life.

To get back in shape (very generic destination), you should create a more specific goal like following an intermittent fasting protocol for a full month. For every goal you set for yourself, you should be as specific and precise as possible. For instance, an example of a well-built goal could be "I am going to lose 10 lbs in one month by following an intermittent fasting protocol".

Measurable goals

In order to be able to track the progress made, your goals should be measurable. "I'm going to follow an intermittent fasting protocol" is a difficult goal to measure and to track compared to "every day I have only an 8 hour window to eat". In practice, you must be able to determine if you have reached your goal or not.

Be realistic when setting up your goals

It is important to evaluate your situation honestly and distinguish realistic goals from unlikely ones. Ask yourself if you have all the tools needed to reach the set goal.

If you don't have the time or interest needed to dedicate many hours to an intermittent fasting protocol every week, this goal is not for you. If this were your case, it will therefore be necessary to choose an alternative path - there are many ways, in fact, to be able to keep yourself in shape without having to follow an intermittent fasting protocol.

At every moment you will have many goals and at different completion stages. You have to decide which are the most important or urgent ones for you. Being committed to achieving too many goals simultaneously will make you feel overwhelmed and will reduce your chances of success. It can be useful to set some main priorities. In this way, when two goals will come into conflict, you will know how to behave. If the choice will fall between completing one or two minority goals or a priority one, you will have no doubt on what to do.

Keep track of the progress made

Writing in a diary allows you to track your progress, both personal and professional and, when you are directed towards a goal, performing an analysis of the steps taken is a great way to keep you motivated. Analyzing your achievements will be a good source of motivation to do better.

Give the right value to the achievement of your goals

Whenever you reach a goal, you should recognize and celebrate your success as it deserves. Reflect on the path that led you to the goal, from the beginning to the end. Evaluate if the goal has satisfied you, evaluate your new skills and knowledge and note if the goal has been reached in full. Once you have reached your goal, just set another one for yourself to keep building on the momentum you have created.

Now that we have seen how to set good goals for a healthier version of you, it is time to analyze how to actually write them down to make sure you have the highest chance of reaching them. After that, we will finally be able to start talking about the most effective intermittent fasting protocols you can follow to lose weight fast.

Chapter 3 - How to Write Down Your Goals for Maximum Results

As we have seen in the previous chapters, a goal is a mental representation of a specific and measurable result that you want to reach through commitment to certain actions. At its base there may be a dream or hope, but unlike dreams a goal is quantifiable. With a well-written goal, you will know what you want to get and how you intend to get it. Writing personal goals can be both incredibly satisfying and widely useful. Some studies have shown that setting goals for your intermittent fasting protocol can help you feel much safer and confident, even when it comes to long-term fasting periods. As the Chinese philosopher Lao Tzu said: "A thousand miles trip starts with a single step". You can start taking the journey that will take you to the desired destination by writing down your personal weight loss goals.

Reflect on what is considered significant

Studies show that when your goals concern something that you consider motivating, you are more likely to reach them. Identify the areas of your life in which you would like to make changes. In this initial phase, it is normal for every area to have rather large borders. Generally, people decide to give themselves goals in terms of self-improvement and physical health. An accurate intermittent fasting protocol can help you move towards these two directions at the same time.

You should start by drafting out your goals on a piece of paper. For example, you may want to make significant changes in areas concerning health and physical well being. Write down this information, specifying what you would like to change.

At this stage you could indicate the goals in vague terms, it is normal. As for health, for example, you could write "improve physical form" or "healthy eating".

Identify your "best self"

Studies suggest that determining which you think is the best possible version of yourself can help you feel more positive and satisfied with your life. No less important, it is a way to understand what are the goals that you really consider significant. Identifying what is the "best yourself as possible" requires two steps. First of all, you have to see yourself in the future, once you reach your goals, and evaluate what are the qualities you need to get to that point.

Imagine a moment in the future when you have become the best possible version of yourself. How will you be? What things will you give more importance to? At this point, it is essential to concentrate on what "yourself" considers important, ignoring the pressures and desires of others.

Imagine the details of this "future you" and think positive. You can think about something that is the "dream of your life", a fundamental stage of your weight loss journey or some other significant result. For example, your best self could be a healthy woman who follows an intermittent fasting protocol with ease. In this case, imagine what you would do. Which intermittent fasting protocol would you follow? How many calories would you eat per day?

Please, put as many details of your best self when writing down your goals. Imagine what qualities your "best self" is using to achieve success. For example, assuming that you are following an intermittent fasting protocol, surely you would know how to meal prep and manage hunger. Those are two skills you just discovered you must develop to improve your health.

Once you have a list of the skills you need to develop, think about which of these qualities you already have. Be honest with yourself, not severe. Then reflect on the qualities you can develop. Imagine ways to be able to develop the habits and skills you need. For example, if you want to follow an intermittent fasting protocol, but you have no knowledge about eating healthy, you can buy a few books about this topic. The beauty of knowledge is that it can be acquired.

Fix priorities for different areas

Once you have filled out a list of areas in which you would like to make changes, you have to put them in order of priority. Trying to improve all aspects of your life at once is likely to end up with you feeling exhausted, running the risk of failing to achieve your goals because they seem impossible.

Divide your goals in three distinct sections:
- General goals
- Second-level goals
- Third-level goals

The first are the most important, because they are the ones who feel more significant to you. Those of the second and third level are relevant, but you do not give them the same value as the general goals. They also tend to be more specific.

An example might be helpful. At the general level you might want to "give priority to your health by following an intermittent fasting protocol". At the second level you may want to "be a good friend, keep the house clean, and be a good parent". At the third level you might want to "Learn to knit or become more efficient at work".

Start narrowing the field

When you have established what the areas you would like to change are and what changes you would like to make, you can start determining the specifications of what you would like to achieve. These specifications will be the basis of your goals. By answering some questions you will be able to identify the who, the what, the when, the where and the results you want to achieve.

Studies carried out suggest that formulating a specific goal not only increases the chances of being able to reach it, but it also helps you feel more happy about the changes it requires.

Determine the who

When you formulate a goal, it is important to determine who is responsible for achieving every sub-goal. Since we are talking about personal goals, it is very likely that the responsible is you. Nevertheless, some goals require the cooperation of others, so it is useful to identify who will be responsible for those parts.

For example, "following an intermittent fasting protocol" is a personal goal that probably only involves you. Otherwise, if your goal is "helping my entire family follow an intermittent fasting protocol", it will also be necessary to contemplate the responsibility of other people.

Determine the what

Asking yourself this question helps you to define the goal, the details and results you want to get. For example, "following an intermittent fasting protocol" is a goal too wide to be manageable. It lacks precision. Reflect on the details of what you want to learn to do. "Follow an intermittent fasting protocol and lose 10lbs in 5 weeks" is more specific.

The more details you can add to the what, the clearer the steps you will have to take to achieve your goal.

Determine the when

One of the key factors of correctly formulating your goals is to divide them in different stages. Knowing when you have to reach every specific step can help you stay on the right track, while giving you the clear feeling of being progressing.

Be realistic in setting the different stages you want to reach. "Losing five pounds by following an intermittent fasting protocol" is not something that can occur from one week to another. Reflect on how long it is really necessary to reach every stage of your plan.

Determine the where

In many cases, it may be useful to identify a certain place where you will reach your goal. For example, if what you are pursuing is following an intermittent fasting protocol three times a week, it is good to decide if you intend to cook at home, buy food on the go or have it delivered at your house. It might seem useless to write down so many details, but trust us when we say that they can make or break your ability to achieve your goals.

Determine the how

This step urges you to imagine how you intend to reach every stage of the process to your goal. This way you will define the structure more precisely and you will have a clear idea of the actions you have to do to complete each phase.

Returning to the example of the intermittent fasting protocol, you will need to choose a meal plan, get the ingredients, have the necessary tools and find the time to prepare your meals in the kitchen.

Determine the why

As mentioned above, the chances of being able to achieve your goal increase proportionately to how significant and motivating it feels. Determining the reason behind your goal helps you understand what is the motivation that drives you to achieve a certain goal.

In our example, you may want to follow an intermittent fasting protocol to feel more attractive and be healthy.

It is important to keep the "why" in mind while you do the actions necessary to achieve your goals. Giving you highly specific goals is useful, but you also need to always have a clear motivation that pushes you when things get difficult.

Write your goals in positive terms

Research shows that you are more likely to reach your goals if you express them in positive terms. In other words, write them considering them something towards which you are moving, not something you want to avoid.

For example, if one of your goals is to follow an intermittent fasting protocol, a motivating way to express it would be "eat only from 6pm to midnight".

On the contrary, "not eat from midnight to 6pm" is not very encouraging or motivating. Words become things, so be careful in what words you decide to use.

Make sure your goals are based on performance

Succeeding certainly requires hard work and a strong motivation, but you must also be sure of setting goals that your commitment allows you to reach. The only thing you can control is your actions, not those of others and not the results.

Focus your goals on the actions you can do yourself, instead of specific results. By conceiving success as a performance process, you will be able to feel that you have remained faithful to the commitment taken even on the occasions when the result is not the one you hoped.

Define your strategy

These are the actions and tactics you intend to use to achieve your goals. Break down the strategy in individual concrete tasks as it makes it even easier to put yourself into practice. Furthermore, it helps you monitor progress. Use the answers you gave the previous questions (what, where, when etc.) to be able to determine what your strategy is.

Determine the time frame

Some goals can be achieved more quickly than others. For example, "following an intermittent fasting protocol for a day" is something you can start doing immediately. For other goals, instead, you will have to sustain a much longer effort.

Divide your plan in individual tasks

Once you have determined what is the destination you need to reach, and in what time period you have to do it, you can divide your strategy into smaller and concrete tasks. In practice you can determine the individual actions you have to do to reach that goal. Give yourself a deadline for each one of them to know if you are respecting your plans.

Divide these smaller steps into even smaller tasks

By now, you will probably have noticed the tendency to break down every plan into smaller ones. There is a good reason to do this: research has proven that specific goals are more likely to be achieved, even when they are complex. The reason is that it can be difficult to act in the best way when you do not know what you need to do.

Lists the specific actions you are already taking towards your goal

It is likely that you are already behaving or acting in the correct direction. For example, if you wish to follow an intermittent fasting protocol, you might already be skipping breakfast.

Try to be the most specific possible when you create this list. You could realize you have already completed the tasks or duties without even noticing it. This is a very useful exercise that can give you the feeling of being progressing towards the goal.

Identify what skills you need to learn and develop

With regard to many goals, it is likely that you have not yet developed all the qualities or habits that are needed to reach them. Reflect on what skills and habits you can already count on that are useful to your goal. The exercise of the "best possible version of yourself" can be useful in this case as well.

Make a plan for today

One of the main causes why women fail to achieve their weight loss goals is that they think they have to start to pursue them tomorrow. Think of something you can do today to start putting a part of your plans into practice, it doesn't matter if it is a very small action. The action you have completed today can be of a preparatory type for those you will have to do in the following days. For example, you may notice that you have to collect information before making a certain meal plan for your intermittent fasting protocol. You could browse the web and learn how to cook those foods in the best way. Even a small achievement like this one will provide you with a good dose of the motivation you need to continue.

Identify the obstacles

No one likes to think about the obstacles that can prevent them from succeeding, but it is essential to identify the difficulties you could meet when developing your plan to reach your weight loss goal. This step is useful to make you find ready in case something goes differently from how you planned it. Identify the potential obstacles and actions you will have to take to overcome them.

Fear is one of the main obstacles women face when starting an intermittent fasting protocol. The fear of not being able to get what you want can prevent you from taking productive steps that would allow you to achieve success. The next section of the chapter will teach you to fight your fears using some specific techniques.

Use visualization

Research has shown that visualization may have significant effects on improving your performance. Often, athletes claim that visualizing is the technique at the base of their successes. There are two types of visualization

- Visualization of the result
- Visualization of the process

If you want to have the highest probability of succeeding, you should combine them both.

Visualizing the result means imagining to reach your goal. As for the exercise of the "best self", the visualized image should be the most specific and detailed possible. Use all your senses to create this mental photograph: imagine who is there with you, what smells you perceive, what you hear, how you're dressed, where you are. At this stage of the process, it could be useful to build a vision board.

Visualizing the process means imagining the steps you need to take to be able to achieve your goal. Think of all the actions you have undertaken. The psychologists define it as "prospective memory". This process can help you believe that the tasks you face are feasible. In some cases you will even have the feeling of having already completed them with good results.

Use the power of positive thinking

Some studies have shown that, instead of concentrating on defects and errors, thinking positively can help you adapt better to situations, to learn more easily and change effortlessly. No matter what your goal is: thinking positive is as effective for maximum level athletes as for women that want to lose weight.

Some studies have even demonstrated that positive and negative thinking affect different areas of the brain. Positive thinking stimulates areas of the brain associated with visual processing, imagination, the ability to have detached views, empathy and motivation.

For example, remind yourself that your goals are positive growth experiences instead of something that forces you to avoid certain foods or abandon your habits.

If you have difficulty reaching your goals, ask the support of friends and family.

Recognize the "false hope syndrome"

This is an expression with which psychologists describe a cycle that is probably not foreign to you, if you have written a list of resolutions for the new year before. This cycle is composed of three parts: 1) fix the goal, 2) be surprised to find out how difficult it is to reach that goal 3) give up on the goal.

The same cycle can intervene when you expect to get immediate results (which often happens with resolutions for the new year). Fixing specific temporal strategies and deadlines will help you fight these unrealistic expectations.

The same can happen when the initial enthusiasm, which is born when establishing your goals, vanishes and the only thing that remains is the work you need to do to reach them. Formulating strategies and dividing them in smaller tasks can help you keep the momentum you need. Whenever you carry out an assignment, even the smallest one, you can (and you will have to) celebrate your success.

Consider false steps as opportunities to learn more about yourself

The studies carried out show that women who know how to learn from their mistakes have a more positive vision regarding the possibility of achieving their goals. Optimism is a vital component of success. When you are confident you are more likely to be able to look forward instead of backwards.

Research has also shown that the number of false steps committed by those who reach success is neither lower nor higher than those who surrender. The only difference is given by how women choose to consider their mistakes.

Stop searching for perfection

Often, the search for perfectionism originates from the fear of being vulnerable. In many cases we have the desire to "be perfect" to avoid having to face a defeat or a "failure", but the truth is that perfectionism cannot protect us from these experiences, which are completely natural for human beings. The only result you would get would be to impose standards that are impossible to reach. Several studies have confirmed that there is a very strong link between perfectionism and unhappiness.

Be grateful for who you are right now

Research has shown that there is a considerable bond between the active practice of gratitude and the ability to reach your goals. Keeping a diary of gratitude is one of the simplest and most effective methods to learn to feel grateful in everyday life.

It is not necessary to write a lot. Even one or two sentences regarding a person or experience for which you feel grateful will raise the desired effect.

The idea of keeping such a diary could seem silly or childish, but the truth is that the more you believe its power, the more you can feel grateful and happy. Leave the skeptical thoughts out of the door.

Savor specific moments, even those apparently less relevant. Do not hurry to transcribe them into the diary. Take all the time to enjoy the experience, thoroughly reflecting on its meaning and reasons that make you feel grateful. The studies conducted on the subject have shown that to write every day is less effective than just doing it a few times a week. The reason could be that we tend to lose sensitivity to positive things over time, so make sure you maximize the effects of this method.

If you follow these goal setting strategies we are sure you are going to have an advantage over those women that just decide to start an intermittent fasting protocol without the right mindset.

Chapter 4 - The Basics of Nutrition

Now that we have talked about the right mindset you need to achieve your weight loss goals, it is time to study the basics of nutrition. In fact, by understanding how foods behave once they enter your body, you will discover the best way to eat while following an intermittent fasting protocol. Remember that our goal is to help you lose weight while staying healthy. You should never sacrifice your long term health to lose weight faster. This has never worked out well and never will.

During the evolution of the species, humans have undergone a variation of the alimentary patterns due to a multiplicity of factors. From its origin mankind is omnivorous, able to consume a wide variety of plant and animal materials. It is even noted that omnivorism goes back in time, uniting sandwiches and little men to this diet, differentiating them from other evolutionary lines. In this sense, already from the origins Homo is assimilated to the omnivorism of chimpanzees and bonobo, and relatively distant from the vegetarianism of orangutans.

During different phases of the paleolithic the various hominin species employed hunting, fishing and harvesting as primary sources of food, alternating to the spontaneous plants the animal proteins, and preceding in the evolutionary history the finding of such proteins through saprophagous behaviors (ethology widely spread in H. habilis). It has been proven that the genus Homo has used fire since the time of the predominance of the species Homo erectus that of the fire made documented use, probably also for preparing and cooking food before consuming it. According to Lewis Binford, the feeding of animal carrions has extended to later genera than habilis, involving the so-called Peking Man.

The use of fire has become documented regularly in the species H. sapiens and H. neanderthalensis. It is hypothesized, on a scientific basis, that an evolutionary engine for H. erectus, the first hominid documented to be able to cook food was formed by obtaining, with cooking, more calories from the diet, decrease the hours dedicated to the feeding overcoming the metabolic limitations that in the other primates have not allowed an encephalization and a neuronal development tied to the size of the brain in proportion to the body size. This, combined with an increasing consumption of animal proteins, documented to be ascribed to the Homo-Australopithecus separation, or H. habilis-H. erectus, would have been a powerful evolutionary impulse.

Nutrition is a multifaceted process that depends on the integrity of the functions, such as the introduction of food into the oral cavity, chewing, swallowing, digestion, intestinal transit, absorption and metabolism of nutrients. Human nutrition corresponds to the conscious consumption of food and drink; it is influenced by biological, relational, psychological, sensory or socio-cultural factors. In some periods of life as a newborn or elderly, as well as for some pathologies, an organism may not be able to feed itself autonomously, but it needs assistance. In this case we speak of «assisted nutrition».

When the organism is fed by ways that bypass the natural mode, an «artificial nutrition» is carried out. The medical sciences (human and veterinary) deal with the modalities of administration by artificial routes in case of pathologies involving the apparatuses interested in the introduction of food.

Now that we have done this quick historical introduction, let's take a look at the basic elements of nutrition. We are talking about carbohydrates, fats and proteins.

Chapter 5 - Carbohydrates

Carbohydrates are the most common source of energy in living organisms, and their digestion requires less water than protein or fat. Proteins and fats are structural components needed for organic tissues and cells, and are also a source of energy for most organisms. Carbohydrates in particular are the largest resource for metabolism. When there is no immediate need for monosaccharides they are often converted into more space-friendly forms, such as polysaccharides. In many animals, including humans, this form of storage is glycogen, located in liver and muscle cells. The plants instead use starch as a reserve. Other polysaccharides such as chitin, which contribute to the formation of the exoskeleton of arthropods, instead play a structural function. Polysaccharides are an important class of biological polymers. Their function in living organisms is usually structural or depository. Starch (a glucose polymer) is used as a polysaccharide of deposition in plants, and is found both in the form of amylose and in the branched form of amylopectin. In animals, the structurally similar glucose polymer is the most densely branched glycogen, sometimes called "animal starch". The properties of glycogen allow it to be metabolized more quickly, which adapts to the active lives of moving animals. The most common forms of glycogen are hepatic glycogen and muscle glycogen. Hepatic glycogen is found in the liver, it is the reserve of sugar and energy in animals and lasts 24 hours. Muscle glycogen is the reserve of sugar used directly by muscle cells without passing through blood circulation. Hepatic glycogen, on the other hand, must be introduced into the bloodstream before it reaches the cells and, in particular, muscle tissue. Glucose is relevant in the production of mucin, a protective biofilm of the liver and intestine. The liver must be in a state of excellent health to operate the synthesis of missing glucose from proteins, as is required in low-carb diets. Cellulose is located in cell walls and other organisms, and is believed to be the most abundant organic molecule on Earth. The chitin structure is similar, it has side chains that contain nitrogen, increasing its strength. It is found in the exoskeletons of arthropods and in the cell walls of some fungi.

Role in nutrition

A completely carbohydrate-free diet can lead to ketosis. However, the brain needs glucose to draw energy from: this glucose can be obtained from the milk of nuts, an amino acid present in proteins and also from the glycerol present in triglycerides. Carbohydrates provide 3.75 kcal per gram, proteins 4 kcal per gram, and fats provide 9 kcal per gram. In the case of proteins, however, this information is misleading as only some of the amino acids can be used to derive energy. Similarly, in humans, only some carbohydrates can provide energy, including many monosaccharides and disaccharides. Other types of carbohydrates can also be digested, but only with the help of intestinal bacteria. Ruminants and termites can even digest cellulose, which is not digestible by other organisms. Complex carbohydrates which cannot be assimilated by man, such as cellulose, hemicellulose and pectin, are an important component of dietary fibre. Carbohydrate-rich foods are bread, pasta, legumes, potatoes, bran, rice and cereals. Most of these foods are rich in starch. The FAO (Food and Agriculture Organization) and the WHO (World Health Organization) recommend to ingest 55-75% of the total energy from carbohydrates, but only 10% from simple sugars. The glycemic index and glycemic load are concepts developed to analyze the behavior of food during digestion. These classify carbohydrate-rich foods based on the speed of their effect on blood glucose level. The insulin index is a similar, more recent classification that classifies food by its effect on blood insulin levels, caused by various macronutrients, especially carbohydrates and certain amino acids present in food. The glycemic index is a measure of how quickly carbohydrates of food are absorbed, while the glycemic load is the measure that determines the impact of a given amount of carbohydrates present in a meal.

When you follow an intermittent fasting protocol, during the fasting hours your body is depleted from its carbohydrates reserves and uses fat to fuel your movements and thoughts. This is what allows you to literally melt fat once you reach the last few hours of your fast. It is a powerful concept inspired by nature and it works incredibly well for women of your age.

Chapter 6 - Proteins

In chemistry, proteins (or protids) are biological macromolecules made up of amino acid chains bound together by a peptide bond (a link between the amino group of one amino acid and the carboxylic group of the other amino acid, created through a condensation reaction with loss of a water molecule). Proteins perform a wide range of functions within living organisms, including catalysis of metabolic reactions, synthesis functions such as DNA replication, response to stimuli, and transport of molecules from one place to another. Proteins differ from each other especially in their sequence of amino acids, which is dictated by the nucleotide sequence preserved in the genes and which usually results in protein folding and a specific three-dimensional structure that determines its activity.

By analogy with other biological macromolecules such as polysaccharides and nucleic acids, proteins form an essential part of living organisms and participate in virtually every process that takes place within cells. Many are part of the category of enzymes, whose function is to catalyze biochemical reactions vital to the metabolism of organisms. Proteins also have structural or mechanical functions, such as actin and myosin in the muscles and proteins that make up the cytoskeleton, which form a structure that allows the cell to be maintained. Others are essential for inter- and intracellular signal transmission, immune response, cell adhesion and cell cycle. Proteins are also necessary elements in animal nutrition, since they cannot synthesize all the amino acids they need and must obtain the essential ones through food. Thanks to the digestion process, the animals break down the proteins ingested in the individual amino acids, which are then used in the metabolism.

Once synthesized in the organism, proteins exist only for a certain period of time and then are degraded and recycled through cellular mechanisms for the protein turnover process. The duration of a protein is measured in terms of half-life and can be very varied. Some may exist for only a few minutes, others up to a few years. However, the average lifespan in mammalian cells is between 1 and 2 days. Abnormal and misfolded proteins can cause instability if they are not degraded more quickly.

Proteins can be purified from other cellular components using a variety of techniques such as ultracentrifugation, precipitation, electrophoresis and chromatography. The advent of genetic engineering has made possible a number of methods to facilitate such purification. Commonly used methods to study protein structure and function include immunohistochemistry, site-specific mutagenesis, X-ray crystallography, nuclear magnetic resonance imaging. The proteins differ mainly for the sequence of the amino acids that compose them, which in turn depends on the nucleotide sequence of the genes that express the synthesis within the cell.

A linear chain of amino acid residues is called "polypeptide" (a chain of several amino acids bound by peptide bonds). A protein generally consists of one or more long polypeptides that may be coordinated with non-peptide groups, called prosthetic groups or cofactors. Short polypeptides, containing less than about 20-30 amino acids, are rarely considered proteins and are commonly called peptides or sometimes oligopeptides. The sequence of amino acids in a protein is defined by the sequence present in a gene, which is encoded in the genetic code. In general, the genetic code specifies 20 standard amino acids. However, in some organisms the code may include selenocysteine (SEC), and in some archaea, pyrrolysine, and finally a 23rd amino acid, N-formylmethionine, a methionine derivative, which initiates protein synthesis of certain bacteria.

Shortly after or even during protein synthesis, protein residues are often chemically modified by post-translational modification, which if present alters physical and chemical properties, bending, stability, activity and ultimately, the function of the protein. Proteins can also work together to achieve a particular function and often associate in stable multiprotein complexes.

Proteins that contain the same type and number of amino acids may differ from the order in which they are located in the structure of the molecule. This aspect is very important because a minimal variation in the sequence of amino acids of a protein (that is in the order in which the various types of amino acids follow each other) can lead to variations in the three-dimensional structure of the macromolecule which can make the protein non-functional. A well-known example is the case of the human hemoglobin beta chain, which in its normal sequence carries a trait formed by the following proteins: valine-histidine-leucine-threonine-proline-glutamic acid-lysine.

Proteins and nutrition

The biological value of a protein identifies its ability to meet the metabolic needs of the body for total amino acids and essential amino acids.

The protein quality varies according to the digestibility of the protein (% digested amount and amount of amino acids absorbed in the gastrointestinal tract) and its composition in essential amino acids.

Foods of animal origin (meat, cold cuts, fish, eggs, milk and dairy products) have high biological quality proteins because they contain all the essential amino acids in adequate quantities and are easy to digest. For this reason they are also called noble proteins or high biological value .

Cereals (bread, pasta, rice, spelt, etc.) and legumes (chickpeas, peas, soya, beans, etc.), being of vegetable origin, contain proteins with reduced biological value and that is of inadequate quality. In fact, on the one hand they are not digestible, on the other they do not contain, or contain in insufficient quantity, some essential amino acids.

To ensure protein completeness, even by consuming foods of vegetable origin, it is essential to combine cereals and legumes by consuming traditional Mediterranean dishes. We are talking about pasta and beans, legume soups with spelt/barley, rice and peas, etc. These foods, consumed together, provide a good quantity and quality of amino acids similar (but not equal) to food of animal origin.

Protein daily requirement

The daily protein requirement of a subject depends on several factors, such as age, sex, body weight, physiological-nutritional status and physical activity.

It should be remembered that the body does not stock protein, so it is important to meet the daily protein requirement ensuring the correct amount of essential amino acids.

Based on the LARN requirements (Reference Nutrient Intake Levels - IV revision 2014) and the quality of the proteins introduced by the American population, it has been calculated, on average, how much protein should be taken by age, sex, and weight. For women over 50 years of age, it is recommended one gram of protein for every pound of body weight. So, if you are 120 lbs, you should get at least 60 grams of proteins per day.

Correct intake of protein

To fully exploit all the potential of proteins, it is necessary to make an optimal use so that they are not "dispersed" because they are used as energy. The energy needed for the human body must come mainly from carbohydrates and fats, so that only a part of the protein is used as energy. Protein foods, in particular of animal origin, must be consumed at main meals, e.g.:

The so-called dissociated diets, which provide only proteins or only carbohydrates, not only do not work, but, without introducing on every meal carbohydrates and fats, proteins are consumed thus establishing a protein-energy malnutrition. Obviously the energy introduced must respect the energy balance. You have to introduce as much as you consume, otherwise the macronutrients in excess (proteins or fats or carbohydrates) are stored in your belly. Another important factor is low-calorie and high-protein diets. The diet of protein alone must be prescribed by the nutritionist doctor who limits its consumption over time and in the quality of nutrients. High-protein diets, or DIY diets can make you quickly lose a few extra pounds, but they also often consume lean-mass proteins (muscles, etc.) and thereby reduce the metabolic capacity of the body so that when you go back to eating normally, you take back that pounds.

Chapter 7 - Fats

Lipids are an important energy reserve for animals and plants, as they are able to release a large amount of calories per unit mass. The caloric value of one gram of lipids is about twice as high as sugar and protein, about 9.46 kcal/g versus 4.15 kcal/g. That's why they are the ideal energy substrate for cells. In a healthy woman of 120lbs, there are about 25lbs of fat. During physical activity lipids are used together with carbohydrates, providing the same amount of energy for medium-low level activities. If physical activity lasts for at least an hour you encounter a depletion of carbohydrate stocks (glycogen) and a corresponding increase in the use of lipids. In addition, food lipids provide essential fatty acids (that is, not synthesized by the body), such as linoleic acids (from which arachidonic acid derives) and linolenic.

In a balanced and healthy diet it is important to limit the consumption of saturated and hydrogenated fats, as they entail an increased cardiovascular risk and prefer, instead, unsaturated fats such as those represented by extra virgin olive oil and those present in fish or oil seeds.

The recommended daily intake varies from 25 % to 35 % of total daily calories. Olive oil contains monounsaturated fats and a whole series of other nutrients such as polyphenols with antioxidant function, vitamin E and anticancer compounds: olive oil is the main food of the Mediterranean diet and must never be missed on your dishes.

Blue fish (salmon, tuna, mackerel, sardines) contains polyunsaturated fats of the omega 3 series. These fats are called essential, because the human body is not able to synthesize them and must be introduced from the outside with food. In recent years, numerous studies have highlighted the vital importance of these lipids, as they have many beneficial effects on our health and even in the prevention of many diseases (premature aging, heart attacks, depression, Alzheimer's, senile dementia, etc.).

Oilseeds are valuable and very useful foods to eat as they contain fat-soluble vitamins, minerals such as magnesium and polyunsaturated essential fats similar to those contained in fish. Almonds, walnuts, hazelnuts, linseed, pumpkin seeds, sunflower seeds, sesame seeds, pistachios, cashews, etc. can be inserted in the daily diet by adding them, for example, to salads or consumed at breakfast or in the snack.

Hydrogenated and trans fats, contained for example in vegetable margarine and in some oils such as rapeseed oil, are to be avoided. In fact, they are harmful to cell membranes and increase LDL cholesterol, blocking even some mitochondrial breathing processes. Unfortunately, these fats are very present in baked and packaged products, so it is important to always read the labels and check their absence.

Chapter 8 - Vitamins

Vitamins, essential organic compounds in many vital processes, are not synthesized by the body, so it is necessary to integrate them through nutrition. The amounts needed are very small (some milligrams or micrograms per day) and for this reason they are considered micronutrients, in contrast to macronutrients (carbohydrates, fats and proteins) that should be taken in much larger amounts, or tens or hundreds of grams a day. Vitamins are divided into fat-soluble and water-soluble vitamins, based on their solubility in fat and water.

Fat-soluble vitamins

Vitamin A refers to a series of compounds that in nature are found in different forms: retinol and retinal acid. Plant precursors of vitamin A are carotenoids, mainly beta-carotene. This vitamin is essential for cell differentiation, foetal development, immune system, skin and vision. Its deficiency causes mainly night blindness, dryness of the cornea and opacization and corneal ulcerations, while its excess induces fetal malformations, liver damage and, in the case of ingestions of very high quantities, cerebral edema and coma. The recommended daily dose corresponds to 6-700 μg. It is contained in milk, butter, cheese, eggs and, in general, in foods containing animal fats. Carotenoids and beta-carotene are present in colored vegetables.

Vitamin D exists in two forms: cholecalciferol, or vitamin D3, and ergocalciferol, or vitamin D2. Cholecalciferol is mainly synthesized by the body and is formed in the skin by the effect of sunlight; ergocalciferol is taken with food. Both of these forms require activation by the kidney and liver that transform them into 25-hydroxy-vitamin D. In this form, vitamin D promotes intestinal calcium absorption, renal phosphorus elimination and the release of calcium from the bone. Vitamin D deficiency causes osteomalacia, a condition in which the mineral component of the bone is reduced with consequent fractures caused by even minimal trauma. Psychological symptoms such as depression and neurological symptoms such as neuromyopathy may be associated. Under normal renal function conditions, the dosage of 25-hydroxy-vitamin D is a good indicator of its state. Vitamin D deficiencies may be due to reduced dietary intake, poor exposure to sunlight, malabsorption (intestinal diseases), kidney and liver failure. The best food sources are milk and its derivatives. The daily intake recommended by Larns (recommended nutrient levels) is dependent on solar exposure. During pregnancy and lactation 10 µg per day are recommended.

Vitamin E includes 8 compounds, 4 belonging to the class of tocopherols and 4 to that of tocotrienols. It is mainly found in vegetable oils, fruits and oilseeds and the daily recommended amount depends on the amount of unsaturated fat intake. The main biological activity of vitamin E is the antioxidant one, which mainly occurs in lipid environments, such as cell membranes and lipoproteins, where there is a need to defend from oxidation the double bonds of unsaturated fatty acids. Deficiency symptoms are extremely rare and manifest with peripheral neuropathy, altered coordination of movements, myopathy and retinopathy. The determination of plasma levels of vitamin E is a good indicator of the adequacy of its intake.

Vitamin K includes a series of compounds belonging to two families: phylloquinone, substances present in the plant kingdom, and menaquinones, produced in the intestine by the bacterial flora. Vitamin K is essential for the synthesis of certain coagulation factors by the liver. Recently, it has been shown its role also in the metabolism of the bone. Vitamin K deficiency leads to a blood clotting deficit with reduced prothrombin time.

Women over 50 are considered adequate contributions between 60 and 80 µg per day. Vitamin K is contained in vegetables, especially in broad-leaved green plants and in the liver.

Water-soluble vitamins

Thiamine, in the form of thiamine pyrophosphate, plays a key role in the metabolism of carbohydrates and branched-chain amino acids. In its absence, glucose is only partially metabolized, resulting in the formation of excess lactic acid. Deficiency of this vitamin causes heart failure, peripheral neuropathy, coma and intellectual and memory impairments. Minor deficits can result in weakness, reduced appetite, and psychological changes. The requirement is about 1-1.2 milligrams per day (0.5 mg per 1000 kcal introduced). In conditions where metabolic activity increases, such as exercise, pregnancy, and certain diseases, the body needs more vitamin B1. Its dosage in the blood is technically complex and is not performed routinely. It is found in food of animal origin (meat, milk and dairy products, eggs), legumes, whole grains and yeast.

Also called riboflavin, vitamin B2 is a substance that becomes part of enzymes involved in energy metabolism. Its deficiency manifests with lesions in the corners of the lips, glossitis and seborrheic dermatitis. The requirement is 1.3-1.6 mg per day. It is present in numerous foods, such as meat, dairy products, eggs, legumes, whole grains, yeast, vegetables.

Niacin can be synthesized by the body from a protein amino acid, tryptophan. Niacin deficiency gives rise to pellagra: the name given to this vitamin, PP or Pellagra Preventing, is to indicate its effectiveness in preventing this disease, which initially manifests itself with skin lesions, then with intestinal disorders (diarrhea) and finally dementia. The recommended daily intake is 14-18 mg. It is mainly found in meats, dairy products, eggs, legumes, whole grains and yeast.

Pyridoxine is a vitamin mainly involved in amino acid metabolism. Its deficiency causes seborrheic dermatitis and microcytic anemia due to reduced synthesis of hemoglobin. The recommended intake is 1.1-1.5 mg per day. It is mainly found in meat, dairy products, eggs, legumes, whole grains and yeast.

Vitamin B12 is involved in many processes, including the synthesis of nucleic acids and the metabolism of amino acids. To be absorbed at the intestinal level, it must bind with the intrinsic factor, a substance produced by the stomach that has the task to protect it in its path from the stomach bottom to the blood flow. Some gastric diseases, as well as surgical removal of the stomach, cause vitamin B12 deficiency. This deficiency manifests with an anemia characterized by increased red blood cell size, increased plasma levels of homocysteine, atrophy of the lingual papillae, glossitis, neurological damage with disorders of coordination and motor skills, even irreversible. Vitamin B12 can be easily measured in the blood. The recommended daily intake is 2 µg. It is made exclusively from animal sources, so vegan diets easily expose its deficiency.

Folates are a group of substances characterized by a chemical structure similar to that of folic acid; some of their functions are similar to those of vitamin B12. They also fall into enzymatic complexes involved in the metabolism of nucleic acids and amino acids. Deficiency occurs with megaloblastic anemia and increased plasma levels of homocysteine. The dose of folate in plasma is a commonly performed survey and is a good indicator of the state of this vitamin. The recommended daily quantity is 200 µg (400 µg in pregnancy). Good sources of folate are fresh vegetables.

Vitamin C consists of ascorbic acids and hydrocarbons. Its function is complex, intervening in redox reactions, in the synthesis of collagen (the most important structural protein of our organism), in the antioxidant activity in the aqueous phase, in the regeneration of vitamin E and glutathione (antioxidant endogenous substance) oxidized. Vitamin C deficiency causes scurvy, a disease characterized by vascular fragility with gingival bleeding, joint bleeding, petechiae (skin spots due to the breaking of small vessels), susceptibility to infection, weakness and apathy. Vitamin C can be measured in plasma, as an index of recent intakes, and in leukocytes, as an index of reserves. It is recommended to take 60 mg per day. It is found mainly in fresh vegetables and large quantities are contained in citrus fruits and kiwis.

Biotin is a vitamin involved in energy metabolism, as a component of mitochondrial enzymes. Its deficiency, rarely observable, manifests with dermatitis, conjunctivitis and alopecia. It is believed that the necessary doses are between 30 and 100 µg per day. Biotin is made from many animal and plant foods and is also synthesized from intestinal bacterial flora.

Chapter 9 - The Secret Formula to Lose Weight

We assume that to lose weight there are no secrets, or miracle diets, or miracle professionals, but there are methods that can be applied differently according to lifestyle and your energy needs. It is also important that constancy and time are our friends. Beyond the type of diet that can be more or less effective, you have to have patience in losing weight. You will see that by losing just 4 lbs you will feel much more deflated and you will be stimulated to continue in the nutritional path.

Caloric Deficit

To understand the meaning of calorie deficit we must first understand the difference between caloric needs and caloric income. The caloric requirement is the energy that our body needs to support all our physiological functions, basal metabolism, physical activities and daily activities. Theoretically, if we consume as many calories as our caloric requirements, we remain constant with weight. At a time when our caloric intake is greater than our energy needs, we increase in weight. On the contrary, if we consume less calories than our energy needs we will create a calorie deficit and therefore lose weight.

All this, however, is not a perfect mathematical equation, as there are mechanisms that tend to adapt the metabolism when we eat more or eat less. This means that when we take a calorie surplus, a part of it is turned into heat, while when we create a calorie deficit not all the deficit will be turned into weight loss, but the metabolism will adapt to the daily calorie restriction. These are the reasons why we don't get fat or lose weight forever. In fact, our organism has mechanisms of adaptation so that it does not succumb to hunger in the short and medium term. Of course, a calorie deficit that lasts for life as well as a calorie excess that lasts for life will lead on the one hand to malnutrition and then to death, on the other to metabolic diseases and over time to death for cardiovascular diseases.

How to calculate your calorie deficit

To calculate your calorie deficit and therefore know how many calories you have to eat to lose weight, you have to know your starting point, that is, you have to know your current daily calorie intake. To do this you must write down everything you eat daily for at least five days, in which at least one of these must be a holiday day where you will eat more than normal. To know the calories consumed daily, you can make use of some well-made and easy to use applications. The most used are Myfitnesspal and Yazio. First, before you start your food diary, weigh yourself and then write down everything you bring to your mouth. Once you know the calories you consume in these five days you'll have to average them. The value obtained is most likely your daily calorie intake.

Many women when they write down everything they eat tend to self-regulate. The consequence of self-regulation is that they will tend to eat less than they previously ate because of the awareness they acquire about their diet. So if you weigh yourself after five days of a food diary, and you've had a slight weight loss, add an extra 5% to your average. This percentage gap is probably what made you lose weight.

How to go in calorie deficit

Once you get the value with your application, you have to figure out how to go into a calorie deficit. The method consists in eliminating enough calories to allow weight loss to happen. Suppose you have a daily caloric intake of 2200kcal. Theoretically to have a weight loss of 500 gr per week you will have to eliminate 500 kcal per day from your current calorie income. Therefore, if you want to lose 500 gr per week you will have to eat 1700kcal per day. Our experience tells us that this calorie cut is relatively sustainable.

In order for the diet to be sustainable and not to allow the metabolism to adapt to the calorie deficit, it must not always be the same, but must change day by day. This means that in a week you will have to eat about 12000 kcal. These calories you can distribute as you want, the important thing is that at the end of the week you will have eaten 12000 kcal. For example, from Monday to Saturday you can eat 1500 kcal and on Sunday 3000 kcal. Of course don't weigh yourself the next Monday as you might have a little more water retention. Wait for next Wednesday. Alternatively you could also do a day of 1500 kcal and a day of 1900 kcal. Basically you can manage the diet however you want, the important thing is that it is from 12 thousand kcal weekly.

This method helps you to follow a more conscious and flexible and less rigid intermittent fasting protocol.

How to build the diet based on the caloric deficit obtained

To build your diet based on the calorie deficit you calculated, with the same application you used to make your food diary, you can build your diet based on your work needs, your schedule and your food tastes. From these choices, however, you will have to have some basic rules, otherwise you will tend to always eat the same foods or the one you prefer. Remember that a diet should also be a healthy food lifestyle that helps you change your wrong habits. Therefore try to eat legumes at least twice a week in the absence of an irritable colon, at least twice a week eggs and prefer white meats to red meats and sausages.

If you can't lose weight then you'll probably have to investigate the reasons for your difficulty. A simple method to stimulate your metabolism is to create a calorie deficit for 4 days a week, and then 3 days of normal calorie diet that in the example case would be 4 days of 1700 kcal and 3 days of 2200kcal.

This method will have to be followed for at least 2 months. Of course, in this way, the weight loss will be slower, but necessary to see an improvement in the efficiency of the metabolism. To improve the efficiency of your metabolism you can keep training as well.

There are also some cases in which you still can not lose weight, despite the metabolic stimulus. In this case it is necessary an impedance to identify the metabolic cell mass and in more serious cases it is necessary to do an indirect colorimetry to understand the proper functioning of the metabolism or alternatively hematologic analysis to identify if there are hormonal problems.

Chapter 10 - Step 1: Activate Your Metabolism

The basal metabolism is the energy spent by the body during the day to satisfy the general functions of the organism, that is the calories spent by the organism for the vital functions such as breathing, circulation, liver functions, brain etc. Basically if you have a basal metabolism of 1300 kcal per day means that at rest for 24 hours without moving you consumed 1300 kcal.

In the basal metabolism the calories spent for the physical activities and the daily activities that we carry out are not included.

The value of basal metabolism is the sum of all the metabolisms of each individual organ. Some organs have a fast metabolism like the heart, the brain, the liver, the kidneys that cover about 60% of the basal metabolism, while other organs have a slower metabolism like the muscle that covers 20% of the basal metabolism. Yes, you understand well: muscles have a slower metabolism, but being widely present in our body expresses a very important share of basal metabolism. This is one of the reasons why the more muscular we are the more the basal metabolism is high.

To increase low basal metabolism you need to understand why the metabolism is slow. The causes can be different both physiological and pathological.

Age is one of the main causes of low metabolism. Of course in this case the decrease is relative and physiological, because it is a lower metabolism than when you are young. With age, after the 50 year mark for women, the lean mass decreases, the muscle decreases, there is a depression of the hormones involved in metabolism such as thyroid hormones and adrenal hormones. With the decrease in lean mass there is also a decrease in mitochondria which are the nuclear power plants of our body that produce energy and allow fat to be burned with greater efficiency. The less mitochondria we have, the less efficient our metabolism will be. Despite this physiological change in metabolism and its efficiency, numerous studies have shown that this process can be slowed down when we do an anaerobic activity that allows us to develop lean mass and musculature. By the time we have more muscle mass we will certainly have more metabolism resulting from this increase. So you can say that metabolism depends a lot on body composition.

Genetics give our metabolism greater slowness or efficiency. There are people who have a more efficient metabolism also based on gene variants (polymorphisms) that help our body to be faster and burn fat more easily (such as the FTO gene or insulin resistance genes PPARG). Genetics is our basis and we can't change it, but we can modulate it through a healthy intermittent fasting protocol and training.

Sedentariness does not help low metabolism. In fact, the movement not only helps to burn more calories, but allows to develop what is called NEAT, that is, the production of heat due to the spontaneous activities that we normally do during the day, such as sweeping, walking, climbing stairs etc. This metabolic component is really important to maintain a high basal metabolic rate.

Thyroid diseases can induce slower metabolism. In fact, not the entire metabolism is motivated by lean mass but at least 20% of metabolism is given by what are called thermogenesis. Thermogenesis are those mechanisms that allow us to produce heat to maintain the internal temperature at about 37°, or to dissipate the excess calories in heat through mitochondria. Thermogenesis is the mechanism that allows your body to produce heat. In fact, thermogenesis in addition to thermoregulation functions help to keep the weight constant. The thyroid hormones in particular the T3 are precisely those that allow you to trigger the fuse for thermogenesis.

Chronic inflammations tend to decrease basal metabolism as inflammatory processes such as autoimmune diseases release inflammatory molecules that "eat" lean mass. Even with metabolic syndrome or insulin resistance, the unregulated diet determines inflammation and therefore a less efficient metabolism.

Sarcopenia, that is the gradual loss of muscle that occurs with menopause and with old age, can lead to a low basal metabolism because you have the loss of those nuclear power plants, mitochondria, which we talked about earlier in addition to the fact that loss of muscle fibers.

Very restrictive diets (below 1000 kcal per day) lasting for many months lead to malnutrition with loss of lean mass, which slows the metabolism.

As we said before, metabolism depends a lot on body composition, in particular on the quantity and quality of our lean mass. The lean mass is not only affected by physical activity but also by the composition of the diet that we have adopted over time. In fact, not only do long-lasting restrictive diets lower metabolic efficiency (in this case metabolic efficiency means the ability to burn calories more easily), but also always do monotone diets such as ketone diets for a long time.

It will probably also happen to you that a diet that made you lose a lot of pounds the first time, the next time does not make you lose as much weight as before. This is because the body records dietary stress. To throw gasoline on the fire are also the diets that eliminate carbohydrates for a long time. Usually these diets are to be done for short periods, but if they are prolonged for more months then the organism takes the carbohydrates it needs from its lean mass, going to deplete the metabolically active mass. As we will see in the next chapters, a healthy intermittent fasting protocol is a safe choice to lose weight for prolonged periods of time.

We speak of low metabolism when through indirect calorimetry for the measurement of metabolism, the value obtained is below the expected value for a woman of that age. Subsequent evaluations can be made with impedance for the evaluation of lean mass and with handgrip for the evaluation of sarcopenia.

Usually the symptoms of a low metabolism are asthenia, changes in the menstrual cycle, hair loss , ease to weight gain or difficulty in losing weight.

What happens to basal metabolism with an intermittent fasting protocol

Before we talk about how to increase basal metabolism, I'd like to talk about what happens to metabolism when we go on a diet.

The decrease in lean mass and fat mass is subjective during a diet, but on average it happens with a proportion of 1 to 3. That is, when for each share of lean mass, we lose 3 shares of fat mass during the diet.

The loss of lean mass occurs with a higher speed when the calorie restriction exceeds a certain threshold. On average, this threshold is 1200 kcal for women and 1500 kcal for men. Going below these values for long periods (about 2-3 months) means stopping weight loss much earlier.

How to increase basal metabolism through an intermittent fasting protocol

To increase the basal metabolism with the diet you have to first bring the question on what is your goal and that is if you want to lose weight however maintaining the efficient metabolism or restore the basal metabolism first without losing weight and then think about losing weight. The importance of choosing these two goals determines the most appropriate food plan.

In case you still want to lose weight but keep your metabolism efficient follow these tips.

- Keep your nitrogen balance positive. This statement means that to maintain lean mass and therefore not lose metabolism, you must take a daily amount of protein with food or supplements that do not allow you to lose lean mass. In this case we recommend making an impedance every 3 weeks to check the amount of lean mass and then calibrate the diet according to its change.

Normally the amount of protein to be taken with food should be 1.5-1.7 grams per kilogram of lean mass.

- Unless you make special diets the diet should not go below 1200 kcal per day for more than 3 months or must be cyclical, that is calories should not always be equal, but at least every 3 days you have to increase your calories by 20% compared to the weekly average.

In order to maintain an active thermogenesis, without a fall in metabolism at least one meal must be protein-based. A meat meal can increase diet-induced thermogenesis by up to 20%.

In case you need to restore an already low metabolism avoid using dietary practices that tend to lower it even more. In such cases then you must first restore it for what is possible. But to do this you have to understand the problem. Here are some ideas for reflection although the causes may be different and sometimes concurrent.

- Avoid for at least 2 months very restrictive diets such as heavily hypocaloric that give little nutrients to the body to restore metabolism.

- Increase your calories gradually by about 200 kcal every 2 weeks until you reach a limit that is your personal limit during which you start to gain weight.

- If you have been on a high carbohydrate diet for more than 3 months, increase your carbohydrates slowly. You have several ways to increase your carbohydrates. The first is to increase carbohydrates gradually daily for example by inserting 30 grams of extra carbohydrates per day or supplement on alternate days carbohydrates with a share of 60 grams total daily (attention how carbohydrates are not meant only pasta and bread). This will tend to stimulate the efficiency of thyroid hormones through thermogenesis.

- Insert a sufficient amount of protein to restructure the lean mass. 3 grams per lbs of lean mass.

During the restructuring period you should keep control of thyroid hormones and also evaluate significant variations of FT3 and FT4 by blood sampling. For there to be an efficiency in transforming the metabolically inactive T4 to T3 than the active hormone, there must be a good amount of glycogen in the muscle and liver anyway.

Therefore meals must still have an adequate amount of carbohydrates that depends a lot from organism to organism because the enzymes that transform T4 into T3 in the liver and muscle are sensitive to the amount of glycogen of the organism and therefore to the amount of carbohydrates that we introduce. For this reason it is not possible to use this method with a ketogenic diet (without carbohydrates), but each meal must be complete with a share of carbohydrates, one of lipids and one of proteins.

Measure your basal metabolism on a monthly basis

Measure your variability through HRV (heart rate variability) through the appropriate instrument, to evaluate the adrenal tone.

To use this method of course you must have a photograph of how much and how you eat. The usual apps like Myfitnesspal or Yazio can help you to know your current situation. Just record with these applications everything you eat for at least 5 days in which it is also included at least one day of diet to know how many calories you eat during the day and how many macronutrients in the form of carbohydrates fat and protein.

If actually your calorie intake is already low i.e. around 1200-1500 kcl daily then for 2 weeks it increases by 200 kcal. Weigh yourself before 2 weeks and after 2 weeks and see if your weight has changed. Of course, always weigh yourself in the same condition. If your weight hasn't changed, then you're doing fine. At this point for another 2 weeks you have to keep the same calories slightly increasing carbohydrates and decrease fat. In particular, you need to increase carbohydrates by 3% and decrease fat by 3%. You can always check these variations with the apps we recommended before.

So, during this journey you will still have to record everything you eat. Once the 4 weeks are completed, the cycle starts again, increasing the calories of 200 kcal for 2 weeks and for another 2 weeks it increases the carbohydrates. When do you have to stop? When you start to see a constant weight gain (no weight swings). At this point you will have found a new balance of weight and energy requirements. When you get to this point, you have to keep this level for another month.

The increase in calories for the restoration of metabolism should not be left alone. To be more effective with this method, you need to increase lean mass at the same time. As we said before, in fact, by increasing lean mass we can also increase the density of mitochondria in our body and the metabolic efficiency. Be careful that if you are a sedentary woman in the first week of exercise you could increase by 1.5-3 lbs due to the increase in muscle volume. This situation is perfectly normal. Physical activity must also be gradual and it is advisable to start with mild aerobic physical activity and then continue with muscle restructuring through anaerobic activity.

Be gentle with yourself in everything you do and your body will respond accordingly.

Chapter 11 - Step 2: Choosing the Intermittent Fasting Protocol

Everyone knows what fasting is but no one pays attention to it when they do it. In fact, fasting is simply when you don't eat, therefore, for most of the time you are fasting. Normally the longest period without eating is between dinner and breakfast, which is about 10-12 hours.

Intermittent fasting is not a diet, but a way in which you can deal with your diet; it involves alternating stages of fasting (or underfeeding) from 16 to 36 hours in stages of feeding and can include any choice of food (paleo, mediterranean, vegan, vegetarian, area and so on).

So nothing special and shocking, it simply adds a few hours to the night fast.

A great advantage of intermittent fasting is that it is ductile. In fact, it does not impose a rigid and pre-established schedule, but leaves the possibility to choose how much to fast and when to fast.

How long it has to last to be effective

Intermittent fasting has no precise duration, you can use it as a method over the long term but only for a few times a week. It is clear that fasting does not mean days or weeks without eating or with a few calories. In that case, you would enter a state of malnutrition. When we talk about intermittent fasting, we speak of fasting periods in terms of hours without eating, not days or weeks.

How often should you do intermittent fasting?

Especially for those who start it is advisable a gradual approach and not suddenly to impose fasting 7 days a week or for an excessive number of hours (e.g. 24-36 hours), it would not be sustainable. It is better to ensure a period of fasting that allows you to eat every day (e.g. 16 hours).

Thus, a good method is to alternate the caloric restriction days to normal feeding days or to impose the restrictive schedule for

4-5 days and leave 2 or 3 days to eat normally (for example during the weekend).

How many meals should you eat

For those who are accustomed to 5 or 6 meals a day it is difficult to go directly to an intermittent fasting protocol that requires many hours without eating. In fact, it is necessary to take the time in which, gradually, you get used to eating less times a day. For example, you can start to eliminate the meals of mid-morning or afternoon.

Once you reach this goal, you can approach intermittent fasting with more ease, where the number of meals is indifferent. The important thing is that the predetermined caloric intake and the feeding/fasting window is maintained.

Intermittent fasting 16/8
This protocol provides for 16 hours of fasting and 8 hours of eating. This does not mean that in those 8 hours it is possible to eat disproportionately and whatever you want, it is important to maintain the calorie deficit and a balanced supply of macronutrients.

In fact, if you exceed the calorie requirement in the 8 hours, despite the fasting of the other hours of the day you will get fat. Fasting sets a new metabolic and hormonal order and, when well calibrated, it is advantageous to burn more fat. In fact, intermittent fasting increases levels of GH, energy expenditure, lipolysis and helps you manage to maintain a good control of hunger.

Blood sugar

In response to hours without nutrition, lower levels of glucose in the blood are established, although clearly to avoid hypoglycemia a hormonal response is activated to maintain adequate levels (such as decreased insulin and increased glucagon and catecholamines). Furthemore, thanks to fasting, there is an increase in stress resistance at the nervous, cardiac, and muscular levels.

Insulin

The positive effect is twofold. There is a decrease in insulin levels and at the same time an increase in insulin sensitivity, although not all subjects respond in the same way and therefore it is good to evaluate this parameter after a couple of weeks.

As for the immune system, there is a decrease in chronic systemic inflammation, throughout the body, but especially at the nervous, adipose and gastrointestinal tract level.

Sleep

Although intermittent fasting imposes a different hormonal pattern than those who do not follow it, there are no repercussions regarding the quality of sleep. Except in the case where the eating window is short and concentrated in the hours before going to sleep.

Contraindications and disadvantages of intermittent fasting

If respected, intermittent fasting itself has no particular disadvantages. In fact, the real problem exists when you do not know the fasting protocol and you do not know how to set it up correctly. Spending days without eating is definitely not the best idea to stay healthy; just think that for example in healthy women after 4 days of fasting there is a decrease of 40-50% of the markers (signal molecules) that indicate the synthesis and maintenance of bone tissue.

Another problem that can occur is not being able to control oneself in the feeding phase, resulting in an excess of food due to stress during fasting; in reality, it is not so frequent. On the other hand, the opposite problem could arise. In fact, having a few hours for meals, you can tend to eat less and therefore you can risk running into an excessive calorie deficit.

During fasting periods all foods that raise insulin levels are excluded. We are not talking only about carbohydrates, but also about proteins and lipids. Therefore water, no-calorie drinks (tea, sugar-free coffee) and micronutrient supplements are allowed.

The calories to be taken depend on what your weekly calorie requirement is and how much deficit you have to maintain. Once you have established this, you can distribute the calories in the week according to the chosen fasting protocol.

Examples of an intermittent fasting protocol

Deciding which time slot to eat and in which to fast depends on your lifestyle: it is certainly easier to skip breakfast or dinner, rather than lunch.

Breakfast vs no breakfast

Skipping breakfast is one of the best options, as it is easier to do, especially for those who are in the morning are not hungry. Whether or not you have breakfast has no negative repercussions on your health, even if a lot of women believe that it is a must for being healthy.

Lunch vs no lunch

Not having lunch is certainly a more difficult option for those who do not have a job with night shifts. In fact, it would mean limiting the hours of meals in the early hours of the morning and late in the evening, for example with breakfast at 6 and dinner after 10pm. These are hours that may not be comfortable, to which is added the stressful thought during the day of having to refrain from eating.

Dinner vs no dinner

Like breakfast, skipping a meal close to the night hours is better because it is more sustainable in time. In fact, the 8 hours in which you can eat thus become the breakfast (for example at 8), the mid-morning snack, lunch, a snack in the early afternoon (by 16).

Every other day

One of the protocols of intermittent fasting involves the intake of a few calories (about 70-80% less than your daily intake) on fasting days, while in the other days you can absorb all the calories you need, even a little more. The goal is to maintain the weekly deficit, easily accessible thanks to the days of (semi)fasting.

It is a good strategy for those women who have the willpower to resist on days with very low caloric intake and not to exceed in uncontrolled binges on days of normo- or light hyper-caloric.

Intermittent fasting to lose weight

There are different reasons why intermittent fasting is a good method to lose weight and promote body composition:

- It allows the decrease of body fat through lipolysis and weight loss
- It increases calorie expenditure because it stimulates mitochondrial decoupling protein
- In a low-calorie diet, it causes less loss of muscle mass

The Myths of Intermittent Fasting

First of all but not obvious: intermittent fasting is not a diet, but a strategy and as such, as well as all nutritional strategies, does not determine what you have to eat during the day.

In addition to this, "fasting" should not be synonymous with tiredness and deprivation of energy. In fact, in the body there are energy reserves that ensure the normal functioning of physiological activities even without food. Furthermore, during the hours of fasting the levels of catecholamines are higher and help to maintain the active state.

Another concept often associated with fasting is that it lowers the metabolism. It is partially true, but only when the calorie intake decrease; it is not a consequence of fasting itself, but rather of the calorie reduction in the long run.

Even for women athletes the intermittent fasting leads to more advantages than disadvantages if well calibrated. For example, considering the more sustainable 16/8 protocol, it might be easy to skip breakfast, train and start feeding hours with a first meal after training.

As for lean mass, fasting in a situation of calorie deficit does not allow excessive muscle damage, which in a situation of catabolism is inevitable. We advise just adapt the protocol to you and your needs to get the best of the training performance, respect the fasting schedule and the intake of the necessary nutrients.

Intermittent fasting and metabolism

During the hours when you don't eat, catabolic reactions prevail, but they are super compensated by anabolic ones during feeding hours.

One of the goals of fasting is to be able to improve the lipid metabolism (and therefore consume more fats) than the carbohydrate one, which is allowed by the many hours without eating in which there is little availability of glucose. To make up for this lack of sugar, cells that can do so (not insulin-dependent) begin to use lipids rather than glucose to derive the necessary energy.

This increases lipid catabolism.

Consequently, precisely for this aspect, intermittent fasting is useful for those who are metabolically inflexible, that is, a woman that exploits more carbohydrates than fat and that does not have a good lipid metabolism.

Intermittent fasting, autophagy and ketosis

Autophagy and ketosis are two biological and physiological mechanisms linked to intermittent fasting. What are they and what are they used for?

Autophagy is a catabolic mechanism that occurs through the lysosomes of the cell components responsible for the destruction of cellular components (for example, of damaged organelles). This process is also driven by calorie restriction and is not selective, concerns the organism in its entirety. In particular, the process promotes the destruction of damaged mitochondria, in the same way as during training, and the possibility of their regeneration, with a strengthening of metabolic activities and a positive impact on health.

Ketosis, on the other hand, is a physiological mechanism used mainly in low-carb/ketogenic diets, but which is also present in intermittent fasting. In fact, after 8-12 hours without food, adaptations to ketosis begin to take place, which involves the formation of ketone bodies, energy substrates for the nervous system when glucose is scarce. We highly recommend you to follow a 16/8 intermittent fasting protocol, as it is the one that has the most benefits and is the easiest to follow for the average woman over 50.

Chapter 12 - How to Follow an Intermittent Fasting Protocol

As we have seen in previous chapters, it can be very frustrating to feel overweight, without considering the associated health risks. You can lose self-confidence and even become a little lazy. To adequately improve health conditions, it is necessary to change diet and choose healthier dishes, controlling the portions. When starting an intermittent fasting protocol, make sure you are getting enough nutrients and avoid restricting your food intake too much. A diet is most effective when accompanied by a healthy lifestyle and the right attitude.

Ask yourself why you want to follow an intermittent fasting protocol

By having all the reasons and goals of your diet clear, you can choose a sensible meal plan that pays off all your efforts. These are only a few of the different reasons why you might want to start an intermittent fasting protocol.

- Manage diabetes. If you are diagnosed with this disease, you need to change your eating habits. The key to living well with such a disorder is to cut back on sugars or cut them out of your diet.
- Reduce the risk of heart disease. By eating foods that lower cholesterol and help you shed excess abdominal fat, you can decrease the likelihood of heart disease.
- Get rid of the pounds accumulated during pregnancy. It is normal to gain weight when pregnant, but once you have given birth, you can decide to regain your silhouette.
- Get ready for summer. Many women go on a diet at the beginning of summer, when they are terrified of wearing a bathing suit. Sometimes small changes in eating style are enough to avoid this fear and not to be caught unprepared for the costume test.

Before starting any intermittent fasting protocol, you should consult your doctor to be sure that it does not adversely affect your health condition. Tell him that you intend to follow an intermittent fasting protocol. Any meal plan below 1200 calories per day can be dangerous. Michelle May, a weight management specialist, argues that "rapid weight loss from drastically reducing calories results in the loss of fluids, fat and muscle mass. Therefore, metabolism slows down and the body needs fewer calories to survive". In addition, the body tends to accumulate a greater amount of body fat, with the risk of developing metabolic syndrome and type 2 diabetes.

Some women use calories to calculate how much food they should eat, others base their intermittent fasting protocol in grams (of proteins, carbohydrates, etc.), others draw up a list of dishes to eat more often and those to eat less often. Decide how you intend to manage your intermittent fasting protocol.

Make sure your intermittent fasting protocol is compatible with the medications you take. You must be sure that your meal plan complies with nutritional guidelines and that it has no contraindications in relation to the drug therapies you are following.

For example, if you are treating hypertension with the ACE inhibitors used, you need to keep your consumption of bananas, oranges and green leafy vegetables under control. If you have been prescribed tetracyclines, you will probably need to avoid dairy products while taking these drugs.

Analyze your current eating habits

Before starting, you need to be aware of your daily diet. So, try to write down what, when and where you eat to get to know your current eating habits.

Put a diary it in the kitchen or near the bed and write down what you consume (dishes, snacks, small "tastings" from other people's dishes, without leaving anything out), the time and place where you eat (in the kitchen, on the sofa, in bed).

Everyone has their own eating habits and "triggers" that lead them to overeat. Awareness is the first step in learning how to properly manage these aspects when adopting a new meal plan. These are some of the most common triggers for women of your age.

- One of the biggest causes of overeating is stress. When we feel out of sorts or anxious, we often try to console ourselves with food. In these cases, you may want to adopt some stress management techniques or stock up on healthier foods to keep this trigger under control.
- It is more difficult to make correct food choices when we are tired. If you have a tendency to gorge on food when

you feel powerless, you probably want to rest and go to the grocery store once you regain your energy.

- If you have a tendency to empty the refrigerator when you are alone, you may want to consider adding some activity or hobby to your meal plan that will keep you busy outside the home and prevent you from eating compulsively.
- If you skip meals when you have a busy day, you'll arrive hungry at dinner time and eat whatever comes your way. In these circumstances, think about including moments in your new diet when you have the opportunity to eat something in your teeth.

Most dieters find it appropriate to count calories, but another overwhelming majority say they don't actually know their calorie needs. We are used to thinking that fewer calories means losing weight more easily, but in reality it is necessary to be aware of the food sources they come from, not just the quantities to be consumed.

Women report that they consume an average of 1800 calories per day. If you are trying to lose weight, your requirements are likely to be even lower, but you should never go below 1200 calories per day, otherwise the body thinks that it is in a state of starvation, and it begins to store fat.

Ask a dietician or personal trainer to help you figure out how many calories you should be taking in daily to lose the extra pounds in a healthy way. Consider how much physical activity you do during the day. Prioritize foods rich in fiber (whole grains) and protein (lean meats). They will help you feel full for longer and provide you with more energy. Avoid "empty" calories that don't give your body the right fuel. Alcohol and foods such as potato chips are great examples of low-nutrient calorie sources.

Follow the guidelines for healthy eating

The Ministry of Health has developed guidelines in the food sector to help the population to eat properly and follow a balanced diet. In other words, you have the ability to know what the right portions are for each food group without indulging in some of them. In addition, you also need to vary your diet by ranging between different food groups, not just eating apples or other types of fruit, for example. Additional important recommendations include: reducing daily calories from added sugars by 10%; decrease daily calories from saturated fat by 10%; consume less than 2,300 mg of sodium per day. Additionally, there are specific instructions regarding the amount of foods you should try to consume each day, including the following ones.

- Eat nine servings of fruit and vegetables a day. A portion of fruit is equivalent to about 150 grams, which is a medium-sized fruit or 2-3 small ones. As for vegetables, one serving corresponds to 250 grams of raw vegetables or 50 grams of salad.

- Eat six servings of grains a day and make sure half of them are whole grains. One serving of cereal is equivalent to a slice of bread or 80 grams of rice or pasta.

- Eat two or three servings of dairy products a day, but try to choose low-fat ones. 240ml of milk equals one serving.

- Eat two or three servings of protein a day. One serving corresponds to 100 grams of meat, or the size of a palm, an egg, 16 grams of peanut butter, 28 grams of nuts and 50 grams of beans.

- Try the "rainbow diet", which is a diet that varies from the point of view of colors (blueberries, red apples, asparagus, etc.). Each color corresponds to different nutrients and vitamins.

Consume more lean protein

The body needs to strengthen muscles, support immunity and keep metabolism fast. To benefit from protein intake without experiencing the disadvantage of consuming fat, opt for leaner sources. Choose skim milk instead of whole milk and lean ground beef or turkey instead of very marbled cuts. Check for hidden fat in meat dishes.

Avoid whole milk derivatives, offal such as liver, fatty and highly marbled meats, ribs, cold cuts, hot dogs dressed with sauces, bacon, fried or breaded meat and egg yolk.

Let yourself be conquered by the fish. Certain types of fish are rich in omega-3 fatty acids, which are substances that can lower the triglyceride index in the blood. You can increase your omega-3 intake by choosing cold-water fish species, such as salmon, mackerel and herring.

Don't underestimate the beans. Also consider peas and lentils. Generally, legumes are excellent protein sources that do not contain cholesterol and have less fat than meat. Try a soy or bean burger, or add some diced tofu to stir-fried veggies or salad.

Consume whole foods

Whole grains are whole grains made up of three parts: germ, bran and endosperm. Therefore, whole foods contain all three components. Unfortunately, carbohydrate foods undergo a refining process that eliminates the bran and germ, resulting in a loss of about 25% of protein and at least 17 key nutrients. To get all the benefits, opt for foods that are labeled in full on the package.

According to some studies, a diet rich in whole grains has numerous benefits, including reducing the risk of heart attacks, heart disease, type 2 diabetes, inflammation, colorectal cancer, gum infections and asthma. They also help maintain a healthy weight, improve carotid artery health and blood pressure. So, don't hesitate to include about 48 grams of whole grains in your daily diet.

Look for them when you shop. 15-20% of food products on supermarket shelves consist of whole grains. So, look for those that carry the "wholemeal" label or look for a product that is made from whole grains or flours.

Diversify the consumption of carbohydrates. There are not only flour and bread, but also pasta, cereals, biscuits, wraps, scones and other products based on wholemeal flour, so read the packaging carefully.

Include healthy fats

Not all fats are bad for your health. In fact, some should definitely be included in your meal plan. Monounsaturated fatty acids (MUFA) and polyunsaturated fatty acids are appropriate because they provide some benefits, such as lowering bad cholesterol (LDL) and increasing good cholesterol (HDL), but they also help stabilize insulin and blood sugar levels.

Foods high in monounsaturated fatty acids include avocado, canola oil, nuts (almonds, cashews, pecans and macadamias, nut butter), olive oil, olives, and peanut oil.

Eliminate trans fats. They are contained in hydrogenated vegetable oils, so you can spot them if you find "hydrogenated oil" written on the labels. They increase bad cholesterol and lower good cholesterol, with the consequent risk of heart disease, cancer, heart attacks and infertility.

Major sources of trans fat include industrially fried and prepackaged foods, especially baked ones.

Beware of products that pretend to be free of trans fat. For example, in the United States, the Food and Drugs Administration (FDA) authorizes "trans fat free" if a particular food contains up to half a gram per serving. Imagine, then, that if consumption is high, every half gram can become an excessive amount. As far as the European Union is concerned, a regulation has not yet been established that regulates the content of trans fats in food products or the related labeling within the Member States. Trans fats are so bad for your health that New York City has passed a law banning their use in restaurants.

Read the labels

By paying attention to the nutritional tables on the packaging, you can stick to a healthy choice of your foods. One very important part of the table is the portion information: it suggests how many portions are contained in each pack and what the nutritional data are for each of them.

It's convenient, fast and easy to eat out or buy ready-made meals. However, you cannot control the preparation of the food or the ingredients used. One of the most effective ways to lose weight is to cook at home. You can choose healthier cooking methods (such as baking instead of frying) and fresh ingredients.

By drawing up a weekly menu, you will be less likely to let the situation get out of hand and order takeaways in the middle of the week. You can make your life easier by preparing healthy dishes to freeze and consume according to your needs.

Try to enjoy cooking. Give yourself a new set of knives or a cute apron. This way, you will find the right motivation to spend more time in the kitchen.

Don't neglect snacks. Good news! You can indulge in a snack while following your intermittent fasting protocol. By eating more snacks, you can speed up your metabolism and help your body burn more calories throughout the day. In fact, a healthy snack also helps reduce hunger and keep you from overeating at mealtimes.

The secret lies in the choice of food. Consume fresh fruits and vegetables, nuts or low-fat dairy products. Try a few slices of cucumber with chickpea hummus for a satisfying afternoon snack.

Keep healthy snacks on hand when you are at work. If you have some toasted almonds in your desk drawer, you will be less likely to go looking for cookies left behind by a colleague on a break.

Season your dishes

If they are appetizing, you won't be able to resist the temptation to eat them. To add flavor to dishes and stay healthy, try dressing them with some sauce. For example, you could pour tomato puree instead of butter over baked potatoes to lower your fat and calorie intake. Moreover, it is also a way to enrich the meal with other vegetables.

If you season chicken, fish and salads with some sauce, you can make your dishes more varied and interesting. Try buying a fresh salsa at the supermarket or make your own.

You can flavor almost any dish by adding spices and herbs. By the way, they are all calorie-free. Try buying parsley, rosemary, or thyme. They will make your chicken, pork or salad recipes more succulent and original.

In addition to the flavor, some ingredients are also good for your health. For example, garlic has anti-inflammatory properties. Use it to season fish or soups - you'll get a healthy and appetizing meal. Turmeric is another fairly used spice that should never be missing in the pantry. Try adding it to salad dressings to add flavor.

Avoid popular intermittent fasting protocol

It can be very tempting to try the latest trend in intermittent fasting protocols. Often, newspapers and television networks report the experiences of famous women who have successfully tried the most popular slimming treatments. However, it is important to remember that not only are they ineffective, they can also have adverse health effects.

Most popular intermittent fasting protocols focus on one food group, such as carbohydrates. On the contrary, a healthy diet involves the intake of different foods, which is a program that includes the intake of all nutrients. Avoid diets that require you to eliminate the consumption of certain categories of foods.

Some crash diets can harm the body, because they promote a very low calorie intake, causing serious health dangers. Rather, get the recommended amount of calories for your build and make healthy choices.

Avoid industrially produced foods. Processed foods and ready meals are rich in substances that should be avoided like sodium, saturated fats and sugars. This does not mean that a fast food hamburger or frozen food will kill you, but they are foods that you should limit.

The Dietary Guidelines for Americans recommend not consuming more than 10% of calories from saturated fat. If you follow a daily diet of 1500 calories, it means that you can eat 15 grams of saturated fat per day. Fast-food burgers contain between 12 and 16 grams.

Stay away from sugary drinks. Sugary drinks, especially soft drinks, promote weight gain and obesity. The calories that we take safely from the straw are always calories and contribute to accumulating pounds, so try to remove or reduce their consumption.

The most thirst-quenching drink is and always has been water. Also, by consuming more of it, you will feel fuller and can decrease the amount of food you consume during meals. You can improve its taste by adding a few slices of lemon, cucumber, mint or other fresh ingredients.

Fruit juice looks healthy, especially if it is 100% pure, but it contains a lot of sugar. Drink it in moderation or add a little water for beneficial nutritional effects with fewer calories. In a study conducted by researchers at Harvard University, the consumption of sugary drinks is linked to 180,000 deaths worldwide per year, including 25,000 in the United States alone. Another study dating back to 2013, conducted by scientists at Imperial College London, found that the risk of type 2 diabetes increases by 22% for every 340g of sweetened drinks consumed daily.

Avoid certain ingredients depending on your health condition

If you have a digestive disorder that prohibits you from taking certain ingredients, read labels carefully and stock up on products that fit your dietary needs. Follow these guidelines and ask your doctor for medical advice before starting an intermittent fasting protocol.

- Celiac disease. Celiac disease is a chronic inflammation of the small intestine caused by intolerance to gluten, a protein found in wheat, rye and barley. Thanks to a greater awareness of the needs of gluten intolerant subjects, it is possible to find various gluten-free products not only in specialized shops, but also in normal supermarkets.

- Hypertension. It is a dangerous disease that precedes heart disease and heart attack. It can be partly managed with a diet rich in fruits, vegetables and lean proteins. The DASH diet - acronym for "Dietary Approaches to Stop Hypertension", or nutritional approach to reduce hypertension - has been shown to lower blood pressure. It is recommended by various health organizations, including the U.S. National Institutes of Health, and has been ranked the best diet of 2012 by the U.S. News and World Report, a US communications company that publishes news, opinion, consumer advice and market analysis.

- Food allergy. If you suspect you have a food allergy, get allergy tests. Eight foods are responsible for 90% of all food allergies: peanuts, nuts, milk, eggs, cereals, soy, fish and shellfish. If you are allergic, read the packaging carefully to avoid products that can trigger allergic reactions.

While you may be tempted to cut your calorie needs drastically and set high expectations to accelerate weight loss, a slow, determined approach will be more effective and easier to maintain.

Change only one meal a day. Instead of suddenly starting an intermittent fasting protocol, try to introduce only one healthier or smaller meal per day. By gradually changing your diet, you will not feel deprived of anything, but you will have time to adjust to the new situation.

Move your body

A proper intermittent fasting protocol allows you to start adopting a healthier lifestyle. However, you will see better results if you also start exercising. According to some studies, combining diet and physical activity results in health benefits and weight loss.

Try to exercise at least an hour a day. You can break it down into steps of a few minutes to make it more manageable. For example, try walking to work and climbing stairs instead of driving and taking the elevator.

Get some rest

If you don't get enough sleep, you are more likely to gain weight. When you can't rest, your body produces more cortisol, the stress hormone, causing you to seek comfort in food rather than encouraging you to make healthier choices.

Try to sleep for 7-9 hours every night. This way, you will tend to have a healthier body weight than when you only sleep 5-6 hours. Avoid using devices that emit blue light (smartphones, tablets, laptops, and televisions) at least half an hour before bed, as they can keep you awake. Try to keep the pace. If you go to bed at the same time every night and wake up at the same time every morning, you will be more active and rested.

Check your progress

To keep track of your improvements, establish a system that allows you to see how you are doing. The food diary you started writing to keep track of old eating habits can be a great tool to know which way you are headed. Compare your progress, temptations, and successes each week.

Enter all the information relating to your new food plan (starting weight, target weight, daily menus) in a software that monitors your evolution. Many programs also offer healthy recipes and provide forums where you can connect with other people who share your goals.

Check your weight every week. It is not only the daily diet that matters, but also what the scales say. Establish a day a week to weigh yourself and write down the results you have achieved.

Set goals that will allow you to improve your health. To have a healthy lifestyle, you need to learn to set realistic goals. Don't make impossible claims, like "lose 7 lbs in a month". Instead, set smaller, more achievable goals. Typically, to lose weight properly, you need to lose 1lbs per week. Set yourself manageable goals, such as working out six days a week. This way, you will be able to accomplish them more easily and you can reward yourself every time you reach a small milestone. Avoid food-based rewards; give yourself a new tracksuit or a pair of sneakers.

Pay attention to food. Nowadays it is very common to eat while watching TV, checking your cell phone or about to go out, but there is a risk of gulping down more than you need. When it's time for lunch or dinner, eliminate all distractions and sit down at the table. Focus on the food in front of you and appreciate its scent, appearance, taste and texture. Put your fork down between bites to give yourself time to chew thoroughly.

Stop once you've reached your goal

Some intermittent fasting protocols are real lifestyles that can be followed continuously, while others are designed to achieve specific goals in a shorter period of time. Many are fine if they last for a while, but in the long run they risk not being healthy.

Pay attention to the "yo-yo" effect. Also known as weight cyclicality, it is the phenomenon in which the cyclical loss and regain of body weight occurs following various diets. It can cause psychological distress, dissatisfaction and binge eating and, over time, damage the cells that line blood vessels, increasing the risk of heart disease.

Ending an intermittent fasting protocol can be a relief, but if you resume your old eating habits, you risk regaining the weight you lost so hard. Instead, try a maintenance program to stay fit.

If you have followed an intermittent fasting protocol based on liquid foods or which has significantly limited calorie intake, you must be careful to gradually reintroduce solid foods into your diet so as not to traumatize the body. Consume homemade soups, fruits and vegetables for a few days before adjusting to a healthy eating routine.

Stay positive and get a healthy picture of your body.

The strength of positive thinking is not a chimera. In fact, it is crucial to eat a balanced diet. It can keep motivation high, but also energy. On the other hand, negative thoughts can promote bad behavior, such as hitting on food to satisfy emotional hunger and skipping workouts.

Don't be negative. Try not to blame yourself if you go wrong and eat pizza instead of something healthier. Instead, get back on track the next day.

Some days it is difficult to feel comfortable in your own skin. It mostly happens if you are constantly surrounded by extraordinarily thin figures of famous people. However, it is very important for general health and well-being to have a positive body image: it increases your self-esteem and predisposes you to make healthy choices.

Focus on the best aspects of your body. If you love your arms, say it when you look in the mirror. Get in the habit of complimenting yourself at least once a day.

Record a thought-provoking sentence or quote when you mirror yourself. By encouraging yourself every day, over time you will be able to develop a more positive body image.

Be kind to yourself

According to some research, if you are more forgiving of yourself, you will be able to get back into shape more easily. When a negative thought comes to you, try to recognize it and then let it go. It really doesn't make sense to blame yourself for missing a session at the gym. It is much more effective to forgive yourself and move on.

Tell someone (or everyone) that you are following an intermittent fasting protocol. By declaring it, you will prepare yourself to successfully carry out your business, because you will take responsibility in front of others. You may also count on the support of family and friends who will encourage you to achieve your goal.

Stick encouraging phrases on the refrigerator. By having wise words that can lift your mood, you will be able to face the most difficult days of your diet.

Don't deprive yourself of everything that makes you feel good. Go to a beauty center, go to the hairdresser, buy a new perfume.

Anything that makes you feel special and pampered can make up for the lack that sometimes creeps in when following an intermittent fasting protocol.

We are sure that if you follow these tips you are going to feel amazing while following your intermittent fasting protocol. At this point you should have all the basic information you need to get started. In the next chapters we are going to dive deeper into specific topics concerning intermittent fasting.

Chapter 13 - Add more Fibers to Your Intermittent Fasting Protocol

The importance of dietary fiber is considerable. Dietary fiber, in fact, has a series of beneficial effects, such that it is an integral part of any balanced diet in the name of health.

Before discussing in detail the functions of dietary fiber and the reasons why it is important, it is necessary to review what exactly dietary fiber is.

What dietary fibers are

In nutrition, it is called dietary fiber, or simply fiber, all that set of organic substances belonging to the category of carbohydrates (with rare exceptions), which the human digestive system, with its digestive enzymes, is unable to digest. and absorb.

Dietary fibers are found mainly in foods that have a plant origin, such as fruit, vegetables, whole grains and legumes. Depending on whether or not it is soluble in aqueous solution, dietary fiber is distinguished, respectively, in: soluble dietary fiber and insoluble dietary fiber.

Soluble fibers

When it is inside the intestinal lumen, soluble dietary fiber becomes, by virtue of its solubility, a viscous gelatinous substance, with chelating properties against macronutrients such as carbohydrates and lipids. Being viscous, soluble fiber slows intestinal transit, causing a sense of fullness.

The main sources of soluble fiber are: legumes, oats, barley, fresh fruit, broccoli and psyllium seeds.

Insoluble fibers

When found in the intestine, insoluble dietary fiber absorbs water, which has the effect of increasing the volume of stool and making it softer. Thanks to the consequences described above, dietary fiber speeds up intestinal transit, interfering with the absorption of nutrients and reducing the time spent in the intestine of toxic substances for the intestinal mucosa.

The main sources of insoluble fiber are: whole grains, green leafy vegetables, courgettes, flax seeds and dried fruit.

Properties and benefits of dietary fibers

Today, with increasing insistence, experts in the wellness sector, such as dieticians, nutritionists, doctors and personal trainers, are keen to emphasize the leading role that dietary fiber plays in a healthy diet.

In fact, dietary fibers have the following benefits.

- They regularize intestinal function, opposing disorders such as constipation, hemorrhoids and diverticulitis;

- They interfere with the absorption of lipids (fatty acids and cholesterol) and carbohydrates (i.e. sugars), making it a very valuable ally in the fight against obesity and diseases caused by failure to control blood sugar, cholesterol and/or triglyceridemia, such as diabetes mellitus, coronary heart disease, atherosclerosis, high cholesterol and hypertriglyceridemia;

- By speeding up intestinal transit, they reduce the time spent in the intestine of toxic substances for the intestinal mucosa, which has a protective effect against colon and rectal cancer;

- They favor the maintenance of an intestinal pH that depresses the growth of that harmful intestinal bacterial flora, whose activity is a source of metabolites known to be associated with the development of colon and rectal tumors; parallel to this, they stimulate the growth of that beneficial intestinal bacterial flora (prebiotic effect), with protective effects on the intestinal mucosa;

- By causing a feeling of fullness, they increase the sense of satiety, which contributes to better control of body weight and the fight against overweight and obesity.

Importance of soluble dietary fibers: the benefits

Soluble fiber is the type of dietary fiber that is the protagonist of the fight against obesity and diseases caused by the lack of control of glycemia, cholesterolemia and triglyceridemia; therefore, the protective action against excess weight and diseases such as diabetes mellitus, coronary heart disease, atherosclerosis, hypercholesterolemia and hypertriglyceridemia depends on the soluble fiber.

Furthermore, soluble fiber is responsible for that improvement in intestinal pH that depresses the growth of harmful bacteria residing in the intestine, whose activity is associated with colon and rectal cancers, and, at the same time, enhances the development of beneficial bacteria, through a prebiotic effect.

Importance of insoluble dietary fiber: the benefits

Insoluble fiber is the type of dietary fiber protagonist of the opposition to disorders characterized by slow intestinal transit (therefore constipation, hemorrhoids and diverticulitis) and to neoplasms that arise from the excessive permanence of toxic substances in the intestine (i.e. colon and rectum).

Are you getting enough fiber while following an intermittent fasting protocol? Probably not. Do you think that to do this it is necessary to eat only salads? Not at all! Read this chapter to know how to consume fibers while following an intermittent fasting protocol.

Find out how much fiber you need

We have already mentioned the importance of keeping a diary dedicated to what you eat each day, including the amount of food you consume. Research each food on the internet and note the fiber it contains. Here are how many fibers you need depending on your age.

- Men under 50: 38 grams of fiber per day.
- Men over 50: 30 grams of fiber per day.
- Women under 50: 25 grams of fiber per day.
- Women over 50: 21 grams of fiber per day.

If you are currently introducing 10 grams per day, don't jump to 21 the next day. You need to give the natural bacteria in the digestive system time to adjust to your new ingestion. The changes should therefore take place within a few weeks.

Start with breakfast

If it's high in fiber, you can probably add 5-10 grams more to your daily diet.

Eat grains with 5 or more grams of fiber per serving. If you can't stop eating your favorite grains, add a few tablespoons of unprocessed wheat bran or mix them with high-fiber grains. If you like toast in the morning, make it with wholemeal or high-fiber bread. Cook muffins containing whole grains or unprocessed wheat bran.

Add fruits such as berries, raisins, or bananas to the grains to increase fiber intake by 1-2 grams. Swap refined white flour for oat or flax flour if you're making pancakes, and you'll add 1-2 grams of fiber per serving.

If you're making pancakes and waffles, use 2/3 of all-purpose flour and 1/3 of wheat bran. Swap quick-cook oats for traditional oats for an additional 2-4 grams of fiber per serving.

Eat the peel of fruits

Incorporating more fruits and vegetables into your diet will bring more fibers in, but only if you eat the peel as well. For example, don't peel apples or potatoes (in the latter case, use the peels to make snacks). You also need to know that by leaving the peel on the potatoes when cooking them, you will get more vitamins and minerals from the pulp. Do not eat the green parts of the peel, they do not taste very good.

Here are a few interesting meal ideas to increase the fiber intake.

- Dry pea soup, a nutrient-dense food: one cup contains 16.3 grams of protein.
- Vegan roast made with nuts and dried peas.
- Sunflower seed cream and dried peas.
- Iraqi shorbat rumman pomegranate soup.
- Dry pea burgers.
- Spinach and dried peas.

Add whole grains or unprocessed wheat bran to stews, salads, vegetables, and baked foods (meatloaf, bread, muffins, cakes, and cookies). You can also use ground flaxseed or coconut flour, two other great sources of fiber.

Eat more whole grains, which are higher in fiber because the husk was not removed during the preparation process. In addition to providing you with more fiber, they will help you lose weight. A diet rich in whole grains changes your body's response to glucose and insulin, which accelerates the breakdown of fat and makes it easier to dispose of subcutaneous fat, which you can see and grasp.

Replace white bread with wholemeal bread. If you can't, make sandwiches using one slice of white bread and one slice of wholemeal bread. Do you prepare it at home? Replace white flour with whole or half whole wheat flour (use a little more yeast or let the dough rise longer and add an extra teaspoon of baking powder for every 2 cups of whole wheat flour).

Eat wholemeal pasta. If you don't like the taste of it, mix it with the refined one or season it more, but don't overdo it. Eat more brown rice or add barley to white rice for more fiber. You will barely taste the barley, especially if you season rice. Eat more beans, which are high in fiber and protein (which are used to build muscle mass).

Just by following these simple tips you will make sure that you get all the fibers you need to keep your body healthy and in shape.

Chapter 14 - Add more Proteins to Your Intermittent Fasting Protocol

As we have seen at the beginning of the book, protein is an essential nutrient for the development and cell growth of the human body, and is important for supporting the body's immune system. Also, adding protein to your intermittent fasting protocol can improve your health and your overall metabolism, especially if you want to lose weight. The amount of protein you should be getting daily varies based on your gender and health goals. To add protein to your diet, you must first determine the ideal amount of protein to consume each day, and then incorporate foods that are higher in protein into your diet. Use this chapter as a guide to determine the daily amount of protein you need, and find out how you can add it to your diet.

Consult your doctor for the ideal daily protein intake. Your doctor can check the correct dose of protein you should be taking each day based on your health status and the goals you want to achieve.

Eat the right amount of protein each day based on your gender. According to the "Dietary Reference Intake" (DRI) system used by health professionals in the United States and Canada, women over 50 should consume 46 gr. of protein per day.

If your goal is to lose weight, increase your daily protein intake. If you intend to add more protein to your diet specifically in order to lose weight, know that you can take up to 120g. of protein per day; however, this dose may vary based on your gender and health status. Replace the meat included in your diet with lean meats. Examples of lean meats that are high in protein are chicken, turkey, fish, or fillet of meat.

Add cottage cheese to your diet. Each 1 cup (236.58 ml) of fresh cottage cheese contains approximately 28 g. of protein. Add fruit or almonds to cottage cheese to enhance the flavor. Add eggs to your diet. You can choose whether to eat only egg whites or whole eggs; the yolk contains about 6.5 gr. of protein.

Throughout the day, snack on nuts, grains, and seeds. Sunflower seeds, chickpeas, edamame beans, unsalted peanuts, and peanut butter are all examples of high-protein foods.

Add yogurt to your diet. Yogurt is generally a high-protein food, especially Greek yogurt, as it is often denser and richer in protein than regular yogurt.

Eat high-protein vegetables. Examples of particularly high-protein vegetables are broccoli, spinach, cauliflower, asparagus, mushrooms, onions and potatoes.
Eat raw vegetables (such as salad), or cook the vegetables by frying or steaming them. These preparation methods will allow the vegetables to keep all the nutrients and proteins intact; boiling vegetables can reduce the amount of nutrients found in them.

If necessary, use protein powders or protein supplements. Protein powders can be added to certain foods or beverages to increase your daily protein intake, especially if you are having trouble meeting your daily protein intake through the foods you already consume.
Add vanilla-flavored protein powder to your coffee, or mix the powder into foods you cook to enhance the flavor, such as pancakes, oatmeal or muffins.

Since there are many different protein powders out there, in the next few pages we are going to tell you how to choose the best brand for your needs.

Protein powder

One way to integrate protein into your diet is through the use of protein powders. The market is full of protein powders, so it's important to know the differences between the products and choose the one that's right for you.

Before adding protein powders to your intermittent fasting protocol, you should know why you want to do it. This way you can choose the protein or combination of proteins that will give you the desired effect.

Add protein powder to build muscle. They are a great way to help with muscle regeneration and building new muscles. If you are training to gain muscle mass, it is a good idea to add them to your diet. However, a supplement should never replace true food sources of protein. It's all about that, supplements. You will need to use them to add extra protein to your diet that cannot be taken with food.Add protein powder to lose weight. Protein increases the feeling of satiety and fullness, limiting your desire to eat. They are also important for maintaining current muscle mass when exercising.

Add protein powders for your overall health. Studies have shown that some proteins help transport bioactives around the body and lower cholesterol. Adding protein powders to a healthy intermittent fasting protocol can help reduce cholesterol, blood pressure, or fat mass faster than a healthy diet without them.

Add protein powder as a dietary supplement. There are many reasons for adding protein powder as a dietary supplement.

- Vegetarians often do not get adequate amounts of protein and need supplements.
- People who have gastric bypass need extra protein due to reduced nutrient absorption.
- People with certain diseases or disorders, such as celiac disease or Crohn's disease, may need extra protein during breakouts due to reduced absorption by the gut.

Protein is stored in the muscles of the body and must be consumed daily or it will be absorbed by the muscles for biological tissue repair. The result would be the reduction of muscle mass and the loss of strength. For this reason, it is recommended that women take the essential amino acids required by the body every day. Most women living in the Western world don't need extra protein because their intermittent fasting protocol is high in protein. This does not mean that using protein powder is bad for your health, but that you will need to plan your diet carefully, including protein powders as a source of nutrition. Research is still ongoing to determine the exact number of proteins for each of us to consume. However, there are recommendations, based on scientific evidence, that everyone can follow.

Get 15% of your daily calories with protein. Each gram of protein contains 4 calories. So in the case of a 2000 calorie diet, you should eat 75g of protein per day. Again, these are values suitable for sedentary people and the minimum quantities necessary to sustain life. Active people are expected to double that percentage, to 30%.

Increase your daily calorie intake from protein by up to 40% (with fats at 30% and carbohydrates at 30%). Extra protein should replace refined carbohydrates (avoid high fructose corn syrup and processed grains). For a healthy adult, this increase shouldn't adversely affect your kidneys if you drink 12 glasses of water a day. By increasing the calories you ingest with protein, you will receive the heart-beneficial effects brought by these nutrients, burn fat and gain lean mass.

Limit your protein intake to 0.8 - 1.25g per 0.5kg of weight per day if you are looking to gain muscle mass and decrease fat mass. If you have any health problems that can affect your kidneys, limit protein to 0.8 per 0.5kg of weight and consult your doctor for frequent blood tests to check your kidney function. The American Diabetes Association makes this recommendation for people with kidney disease or diabetes. Take note of the proteins you ingest with a food diary.

Chapter 15 - Add more Fruits to Your Intermittent Fasting Protocol

Eating healthily is a very important part of a healthy intermittent fasting protocol. Fruit is essential to our intermittent fasting protocol because it contains many vitamins, minerals, carbohydrates and fiber. Here are some easy-to-follow tips for getting more fruit into your intermittent fasting protocol and improving your overall well-being.

Eating fruit on a daily basis can help you maintain a healthy weight and reduce the risk of heart disease, stroke, and some forms of cancer. In addition, fruit contains a large variety of vitamins, minerals, carbohydrates and fiber. Hence, eating the right fruit combinations brings significant benefits. For example, an apple contains a lot of fiber but little vitamin C; But if you add an orange and a few strawberries, you'll get all the vitamin C you need for the day.

Eat five servings of fruit a day if your intermittent fasting protocol allows for it

Many countries have adopted national or regional programs to encourage people to eat at least five servings of fruit and vegetables a day. One glass of fruit juice counts as one serving, but drinking five will always count as one serving. If a third of your diet consists of fruits and vegetables, you are well on your way to a healthy diet.

Adding sliced banana to cereal or dehydrated fruit to oatmeal, or making a fresh fruit salad are all great ways to liven up your breakfast. A handful of blueberries and raspberries can be of great benefit. In fact, in addition to the usual benefits offered by fruit, they also contain antioxidants that protect against DNA damage. These include slowing down the skin aging process and preventing sun damage to the skin; a good start to any day.

Use fruit to snack on

Fruit is the perfect food to consume on the go, and can easily replace cookies, cakes and chocolate when snacking. High-fat, high-sugar snacks contain few essential vitamins and minerals, as well as low fiber, and can lead to poor digestion. So, keep some fruit in your car, purse or on your desk at work, to overcome those energy drops that hit you in the mid-morning or mid-afternoon.

Most food manufacturers enthusiastically insist on the fruit content in their food, to make you think it is a great food. Be careful, though. In fact, not everything that has the word "fruit" in its name is what it seems. Remember to check the fat and sugar content in frozen fruit desserts. Canned fruit in fruit juice is usually fine, but beware of canned fruit in syrup, which may be full of sugar. Try to eat five servings of fruit a day for a week. You will see how good it makes you feel.

Eat your favorite fruit within 20 minutes of waking up. During sleep, your body fasts for nearly eight hours. Eating fruit within 20 minutes of waking up rehydrates your body and provides it with low-glycemic carbohydrates that keep your metabolism going throughout the day.

Chapter 16 - How to Properly Integrate Vitamin B12 During an Intermittent Fasting Protocol

Vitamin B12, also known as cobalamin, is one of the water-soluble B vitamins. Others include folic acid, biotin, niacin, thiamin, riboflavin, vitamin B5 (pantothenic acid), and vitamin B6. All B vitamins play a fundamental role in the production of energy and for this purpose B12 plays an even more important role, which also extends to the production of red blood cells and the proper functioning of the metabolism and the central nervous system. In the next few pages we are going to tell you how to supplement vitamin B12 during an intermittent fasting protocol.

Eat quality seafood

One of the best ways to integrate B12 into your intermittent fasting protocol is to eat seafood. For example, lobster, shellfish and especially clams contain a high amount of vitamin B12. Fish, such as trout, salmon, tuna, and haddock, are also excellent sources of B12. An 85g serving of seafood contains nearly 400% of the daily cobalamin requirement, while an 85g serving of clams far exceeds the daily allowance.

Both meat and offal of beef, such as liver, contain a lot of B12 as well. Pork is also an excellent source of this vitamin. On average, one slice of beef liver contains 2800% of the recommended daily requirement of vitamin B12. Some meat replacement foods such as tofu are fortified with vitamin B12. Consider this option if you are vegetarian or vegan and check the product label for the amount of B12 it contains.

White meats also provide B12, as do eggs. Two cooked eggs contribute greatly to the daily cobalamin requirement.

Do not forget dairy products

To increase your B12 intake, include dairy products such as yogurt, milk and cheese in your intermittent fasting protocol. Some types of plant-based milk are also fortified with this vitamin.

A snack of 250g of low-fat fruit yogurt gives you half your daily B12 requirement.

Try whole grains

Many breakfast cereals are high in vitamin B12. By combining fortified cereals, eggs and milk at the first meal of the day, you will be able to take the recommended daily dose of cobalamin from the moment you wake up.

For example, a bowl (just over 40g) of low-fat muesli with raisins contains 10mcg of vitamin B12, which is 417% of the recommended daily allowance.

Whole grains are a great way for vegans and vegetarians to get B12, since plant-based foods don't contain high levels of this vitamin.

Yeast products and nutritional yeast are excellent sources of vitamin B12. To increase your intake, you can add nutritional yeast to any dish, from cereals to smoothies to evening meals. 5 g of nutritional yeast fortified with vitamin B12 contains more than twice the daily dose of this vitamin.

Take a vitamin B12-only supplement

You can also buy a vitamin B12 supplement in pills. Cobalamin is best absorbed along with other vitamins. Therefore, take it with B6, magnesium, niacin, or riboflavin. In order to get a B12 supplement, you can ask your doctor for a prescription. They may advise you to take this vitamin in the form of an injection or gel.

The recommended daily dose to stay healthy is 2.4 mcg for women over the age of 50. Pregnant and breastfeeding women should take 2.8 mcg.

It is also essential for children, but their needs may be lower than the aforementioned values. The amount needed varies according to age: 9 to 13 years equals 1.8 mcg, 4 to 8 years 1.2 mcg, 1 to 3 years 0.9 mcg, 7 to 12 months 0.5 mcg and from 0 to 6 months at 0.4 mcg.

If you are vegan or vegetarian you should keep the level of this vitamin under strict control. Some women who follow a vegetarian or vegan intermittent fasting protocol may experience a deficiency of vitamin B12, because one of the main sources of vitamin B12 is made up of foods of animal origin. Cobalamin can be obtained through the consumption of fortified cereals. Try eating 3-4 servings a day of B12-enriched foods.

Symptoms of vitamin B12 deficiency

A cobalamin deficiency leads to exhaustion, weakness, diarrhea, constipation, decreased appetite and weight loss. There are also other symptoms produced by B12 deficiency on the nervous system, which include numbness and tingling in the hands and feet, balance problems, confusion, depression, behavioral changes, irritation of the mouth or tongue, and bleeding of the gums. The likelihood of B12 deficiency increases with age, so be careful if you are a woman over 50.

This problem affects women who suffer from atrophic gastritis, pernicious anemia, Crohn's disease, celiac disease, or immune system disorders, such as Graves' disease or lupus. It also occurs in women undergoing partial surgical removal of the stomach and small intestine and in people who drink a lot. Prolonged use of heartburn medications can also cause a vitamin B12 deficiency.

Before taking a vitamin B12 supplement you should talk to your doctor, especially if you are on drug therapy. Taking cobalamin does not involve risks. In fact, in the medical literature there are no toxic or side effects reported. However it could interact with some classes of drugs used in the treatment of gastroesophageal reflux and peptic ulcer. The drugs used to treat these conditions decrease the absorption of vitamin B12. Furthermore, some drugs used to treat diabetes and cholesterol can also reduce its absorption.

If you are taking any of these medications, ask your doctor if you need to increase your B12 intake.

If you have any symptoms of vitamin B12 deficiency, you should see your doctor for a diagnosis. Symptoms of insufficient cobalamin intake can be related to various ailments that need to be diagnosed by your doctor.

If you have been diagnosed with vitamin B12 deficiency, visit your doctor regularly and follow their advice regarding a correct vitamin B12 supplementation.

If you follow these instructions, you will have no issues during your intermittent fasting protocol, even if you are a vegan or vegetarian.

Chapter 17 - How Vitamins Can Improve Your Intermittent Fasting Protocol

Vitamins and minerals perform several important tasks for the body and are essential for maintaining good health while following an intermittent fasting protocol. Most of the need for these elements is met with food and a balanced diet. In addition to helping you take the recommended daily amount, vitamin and mineral supplements also help you lose weight, but you still need to follow an appropriate and balanced diet plan, as well as exercise regularly.

Ask a doctor for professional advice

Before taking any over-the-counter drugs (or supplements), you must speak to a doctor. In fact, food supplements are not always safe for all people.

Although vitamin, mineral and herbal supplements are subjected to careful checks by the Ministry of Health, they are commercially available without a prescription and anyone can buy any kind. Therefore, it is important to receive the right advice and warnings from the doctor, before starting to take any type of supplement, to avoid unpleasant side effects.

Contact your doctor when you think you want to start vitamin treatment so that you know which one is most appropriate for you. Tell them about the goal you want to achieve with this treatment and ask them if there are other possible solutions besides taking vitamins.

If you want to ask your doctor about the supplements you have already purchased, remember to tell them the brand, the type of vitamin and the format (these are on the package label), as well as the appropriate dosage. This information helps your doctor determine if it is a suitable product for your specific needs.

Read the label

Since there are countless products on the market (not always of certain origin), you need to be aware of what you ingest when taking supplements. Check carefully what you decide to take.

Read the directions for all vitamins. For example, if you are looking for a vitamin D supplement, choose a product that clearly says "vitamin D", then read the label to know all the ingredients, so you know the format and all the ingredients. other excipients present. Make sure other substances are also safe for you.

Check the size of the tablet and the dosage of the active ingredient. Nutritional values should also be included in the label. The recommended posology (for example, 2 tablets) and the amount of active substance contained in each dose (for example, 30 mg) should be indicated. Make sure you know precisely the appropriate dosage for your needs and the correct amount of active ingredients contained in the tablets. Do not take more than the recommended daily amount.

Like prescription drugs, many over-the-counter supplements can also have contraindications. Check for any adverse effects on the label and search online for more information if needed.

Take vitamin D supplements

Studies have shown that people who regularly take this dietary supplement (and were previously deficient in it) while following an intermittent fasting protocol lose more weight than those who do not.

Vitamin D deficiency is a major nutritional deficiency, affecting approximately 500 million women worldwide. The side effects of the deficiency of this important substance are many and include: increased mortality, cancer, metabolic disorders, diseases of the skeletal system, heart problems and infections.

Currently, the recommended daily dosage is 400 IU. However, more recent studies recommend taking up to 2000 IU per day if you are following an intermittent fasting protocol.

Vitamin D is fat-soluble, which means that it accumulates in the adipose layer of the body and can remain in the body for up to 3-6 months. You have to be careful not to take too much, as if it is present in the body in excessive quantities, it becomes toxic and can no longer be eliminated from the body.

Vitamin D is present in few and rare food sources. However, you can find it in the following foods: cod liver oil, fortified milk and orange juice, salmon, beef liver, eggs and swordfish.

Take calcium supplements

Some studies have found that calcium, combined with vitamin D, helps you lose weight. In fact, it has been found that taking large amounts of calcium discourages the accumulation of fat in the cells; in addition, it can bind to some fats in foods, preventing the body from absorbing them.

The recommended daily dosage is 1000-1200 mg. However, you should divide this amount into 500 mg doses, as the body cannot absorb more at a time.

Recent research has found that higher calcium levels can cause heart disease and harden arteries. Pay attention to the total amount you take in through the supplements and foods you eat.

The best food sources are dairy products, dark leafy vegetables, broccoli and almonds.

Take magnesium

It is an important mineral that stimulates over 300 chemical reactions in the body. Studies have shown that, in addition to these functions, it also promotes weight loss.

Magnesium plays an important role in many metabolic functions, but it has been found to improve fasting glucose and insulin levels, thereby helping to regulate weight. A deficiency in this mineral can lead to irritability, muscle weakness and arrhythmia. The recommended daily dosage is 350 mg. Take one or two tablets throughout the day. The best food sources are dairy products, beans, nuts, fish and seafood.

The role of probiotics

Although not considered vitamins or minerals, these are supplements that have been shown to be effective in losing fat and maintaining optimal weight.

Probiotics are "good" bacteria that are alive and present in various points of the gastrointestinal tract. They are ingested through food and drink; their purpose is to strengthen the immune system, as well as prevent or manage constipation and diarrhea.

Several studies have found that consuming various types of "good" bacteria and enriching the intestinal flora are two aspects associated with weight loss and maintaining a "healthier" weight.

If you want to include these supplements in your diet, get ones that contain at least 5 billion CFU (colony forming units) per serving.

You can also eat foods that are rich in it, such as yogurt with active cultures or yogurt to drink, sauerkraut, miso, and tempeh.

Choline supplements

Studies have shown that it helps reduce weight and overall body mass. Choline does not fall into the category of vitamins or minerals, but it is an essential nutrient that acts on metabolism, lipid transport and hormone synthesis.

The recommended daily dosage for a woman over 50 following an intermittent fasting protocol is around 400-500 mg. However, specific choline supplements usually contain about 13% of the active ingredient, but generic ones that contain 3500-4000 mg of phosphatidylcholine (the lead group contains choline) are just as safe.

Among the best food sources of choline are beef liver, eggs, wheat germ, scallops and salmon.

Chapter 18 - The Detoxifying Power of Vitamin C

Vitamin C is one of the most important vitamins for the body; you can get it through your diet by eating foods such as oranges, red peppers, cabbage, broccoli and strawberries. You can also take it in large quantities through powdered supplements to mix with water (or other drinks), as it is believed to be able to relieve ailments such as stress, various diseases and hormonal imbalances. Before you cleanse yourself with this method, however, you need to take precautions and talk to your doctor to evaluate the risks and potential benefits. An abundant intake of vitamin C is not safe for anyone and caution should be taken. However, if you have chosen this option, set up and complete the process within two to three hours; if you experience any complications during cleansing, contact your doctor immediately.

Talk to your doctor if you have irritable bowel syndrome (IBS) or hemochromatosis. If you have IBS or an iron deficiency such as hemochromatosis, you must seek the advice of the doctor before deciding to take a large amount of vitamin C because, if you proceed on your own, these diseases can worsen in the presence of high amounts of acid. ascorbic; your doctor can recommend a specific dosage taking into account your health condition. [1]

You should also avoid this vitamin if you have kidney disease or are concerned that you are allergic to ascorbic acid.

Do not take more than 3000 mg per day. Higher dosages can cause blood clots, kidney stones, digestive problems and other heart-related ailments; you don't have to risk overdosing by taking too much at once. [2]

Doses greater than 2000 mg per day can cause cramps, chest pain, dizziness, diarrhea, fatigue, heartburn and intestinal problems; if you are concerned about these symptoms, consult your doctor before taking vitamin C.

If you are pregnant or breastfeeding, you must be especially careful in consuming this vitamin, as in high doses it can cause hypertension; you must always speak to the gynecologist to find out if it is safe for you, for the baby and not to proceed if you do not have his consent.

Tell your doctor if you have vomiting or diarrhea when you cleanse with vitamin C. If you feel really sick, vomit or have diarrhea when starting treatment, you may be allergic or intolerant to the active ingredient stop taking it immediately and contact your doctor right away. [3]

If you experience a feeling of general discomfort or lightheadedness that does not go away after an hour of starting the process, stop and see your doctor.

Look for buffered vitamin C. Pure powder can be aggressive to the stomach and cause ailments such as heartburn and inflammation. Preferably look for the buffered form, which also contains minerals such as calcium, magnesium and zinc and which is gentler on the digestive system. [4]

You can get it online or in health food stores.

Take powdered ascorbic acid. It is an alternative and contains sodium bicarbonate in addition to the vitamin; this extra ingredient regulates the water intake and facilitates the digestion of vitamin C. [5]

You can look for it online and in health food stores.

Have plenty of filtered or purified water available. You need it to dissolve the vitamin C powder; you have to drink a lot of it during purification to help the substance travel throughout the body and stimulate defecation. [6]

You must drink at least 5 or 6 glasses of water during the procedure, after which you can drink as many to recover from detox.

Organize yourself not to carry out any demanding activities during the treatment. The whole procedure can generally last from two to six hours, depending on the time it takes for the vitamin to travel throughout the body. Do not schedule outings during this time, as you will need to have easy access to the bathroom to expel the water and vitamin C powder.

Start the treatment immediately in the morning. Proceed as soon as you get up and before breakfast; in this way, the body can absorb the precious vitamin. [8]

Take 1000 mg of vitamin C dissolved in water every hour. Add this dose of vitamin C powder (in buffered form or ascorbic acid) to half a glass of drinking water, mix with a spoon and sip. [9]

If you don't like the flavor of the vitamin powder, you can add some fruit juice with no added sweeteners.

Repeat the treatment until you start producing watery stools. Continue drinking 1000 mg of powdered vitamin C dissolved in half a glass of water every hour; proceed for an hour or two or until you feel the need to go to the bathroom. Check for watery stools this is a sign that you are cleansing your body with this substance. [10]

It takes a few hours for the intestines to start emptying; be patient; you may need to go to the bathroom within 2-4 hours of starting treatment.

Note the times you take the vitamin during the process. Make sure you keep track of the frequency and hourly dosage; that way, you know your vitamin intake for sure and make sure you don't overdo it. [11]

Also take note of when you make liquid stools to better understand how much vitamin you need to detoxify the body, especially if you plan to repeat the treatment in the future.

Consume liquid meals during the procedure. Cleansing leads to better results if you don't eat large amounts of solid foods; opt for fluid foods, such as soups or broths, so as not to create an upset stomach. Continue like this for the 2-4 hours of treatment and gradually return to solid foods when finished. [12]

Drink plenty of water during your cleanse to help the vitamin pass through the digestive tract.

Insert solid foods like rice, quinoa, and cooked vegetables after the "cleanup" is done. After a couple of days, you can switch to more consistency proteins like fish, tofu, beef, and chicken.

Gradually reduce your vitamin intake. Once your body is cleansed, take a smaller dose of the substance daily for 4-5 days; continue in this way until you reach less than 1000 mg / day. [13]

This gradual decrease guarantees the adaptation of the organism to this change and prevents the purification from having negative effects on the intestine.

You may still notice some water in the stool during this phase, but the situation should normalize when you reach a dosage of 1000mg.

Repeat the cleanse every four months or when you start feeling unhealthy. If you have a chronic flu or cold symptoms, follow the treatment every four months or so, sticking to the first-time dosages for best results. [14]

You can also take 50-100 mg of vitamin C regularly to stay healthy; take it first thing in the morning, even before breakfast.

Chapter 19 - How to Choose the Right Intermittent Fasting Protocol for You

As we have seen, there is a big difference between an intermittent fasting protocol and a diet. In fact, an intermittent fasting protocol is an eating strategy that can be implemented to maximize the weight loss effects of a given diet. However, nowadays there are a lot of different diets and it could be difficult for the average woman to choose the best one for her. In this chapter we are going to examine the most common diets out there to identify which one is the best one for you to implement using an intermittent fasting protocol.

There are dozens of diets in the world, from those that are really smart and in most cases effective, to those that seem to have been invented from scratch and that are useless. In this chapter we will analyze 12 of the most popular diets, ranging from the most restrictive slimming treatments (in terms of calories and food groups), to nutritional styles based on a certain scheme (in which it is necessary to change the times and the way of eating), up to crash diets (useful when you need to quickly lose a lot of pounds). In fact, by having all the necessary information, you can choose the diet that best suits your needs and your intermittent fasting protocol.

Low-calorie diet

It is among the easiest to follow. All you need to do is decrease your calorie intake. In fact, the less you eat, the sooner you lose weight. The assumption behind this eating style is that fewer calories help you lose weight. That said, be careful not to drop below 1200 calories per day.

Advantages. you can eat whatever you want, the important thing is to control the portions. All food packages sold at the supermarket are equipped with a nutritional table. Also, in many restaurants you can find low calorie dishes. In short, it is not difficult to follow it and to integrate it into an intermittent fasting protocol.

Disadvantages. It requires some calculation and some effort, because you will have to keep track of everything you eat and drink, although it should be remembered that technology makes it easier for you. Also, if it is very restrictive, consider that you will not feel full; you may also complain of nausea and dizziness. As if that weren't enough, you'll have a hard time maintaining your weight once you start eating normally again.

Who should follow this diet? If you are determined and have no problem carrying pen and paper with you (or use an app every time you put something under your teeth), this is the diet for you. It is ideal for those women who do not have a large budget and are full of commitments. It is not recommended for those who tend to snack on a lot and for people who hate to constantly monitor everything they eat and drink.

Low-carb diet

It is able to accelerate weight loss, but it is not suitable for everyone. If you follow it, you need to prioritize the consumption of protein and fat (those who support it say that fat is good), so you will eat a lot of meat, cheese, eggs, vegetables, nuts and nothing else. The assumption behind this type of diet is that, when the body has no carbohydrates to burn, it enters a state of ketosis which leads it to directly consume fats (which is why taking them is very important).

Advantages. It is quite easy to follow and allows you to eat many tasty, often fatty foods (such as meat, cheese, etc.), which are prohibited in other diets. There is no calorie restriction, so if it's done right you will rarely feel the pangs of hunger.

Disadvantages. During the initial period (two weeks), people who follow it often feel bad. However, this is a physiological response which passes quickly. Afterwards you feel full of energy, you see an improvement in health and you lose weight. Furthermore, it may be difficult to comply with it because many foods are prohibited. Finally, it can get monotonous, especially if you're not very creative in the kitchen.

Who should follow it? If you know how to cook or are an expert in grilling, you will have no difficulty. It is also ideal for those who do not get bored of always eating the same dishes. However, it is not very suitable for those who love sweets and are not a lover of meat.

The South Beach diet

This diet is similar to the Atkins diet, in fact it eliminates the consumption of saturated fats and certain carbohydrates. Due to its characteristics it is slightly different and some find it more manageable (because the introduction of some carbohydrates is allowed, especially in the second phase).

However, if you are on a low-carb diet, you should take at least 20g per day.

Low-fat diet

In this case, you don't have to eliminate calories and carbohydrates, but fat. It is an eating style that involves some health risks because it excludes essential fatty acids, which are important for the proper functioning of the body. The only fats that are bad for you are trans fats. In short, this diet helps you lose weight because it allows you to take in more calories, proteins and carbohydrates, while restricting the intake of fats.

Advantages. It is quite easy to follow and favors the consumption of fruit and vegetables. Also, in the supermarket you can find numerous low-fat products and avoid those that are notoriously fatty, such as sweets, cakes, cheese, red meat, etc.

Disadvantages. The main disadvantage of this diet is that a low-fat food can contain sugars and salt, substances that are equally harmful to the body, if not even less healthy. Certain lipids are good for your health and there is a risk that the body will want more carbohydrates to fill the gap left by the fat deficit.

Who should follow it? Try it if you like fruits, vegetables, whole grains and lean meats. Discard it if you are a lover of red meats and cheeses, want a meal plan that doesn't involve complications, or are looking for a quick way to lose weight.

Vegan and vegetarian diet

The vegetarian diet prohibits the consumption of meat, while the vegan diet involves the elimination of any product of animal origin (eggs, milk, etc.). That said, there are numerous variations of these two food choices. In fact, there are the flexitarians, who occasionally indulge in meat; the pescetarians, who only include the consumption of fish among their meats; ovo-vegetarians, who admit indirect animal products such as eggs. In general, they are all low-calorie, low-fat, and nutrient-rich diets.

Benefits. This type of diet allows you to lower cholesterol and blood pressure. Most vegetarians and vegans eat a lot of fruits and vegetables, which are ideal for staying healthy. It is not necessary to count calories and sweets are not prohibited. Furthermore, from an ethical point of view they are two diets respectful of animal life.

Disadvantages. You have to be careful. The organism needs proteins that vegetables often do not offer. Being vegan doesn't mean being healthy. Plus, it doesn't necessarily mean you will lose weight (in fact, a vegetarian could technically eat a whole tray of sweets).

Who should follow these diets? Try them if you don't like meat, if you are a good cook (you will have to modify the recipes to meet your dietary needs) and you don't have a tight budget (fresh products can be expensive). Avoid them if you've always been a meat lover and don't want to have complications when cooking or going out to eat.

Glycemic index diet

It is a system that is attentive to foods that can raise blood sugar levels. The higher the potential of a food to raise blood sugar (on a scale of 1 to 100), the less it is considered healthy. A diet like this makes you avoid anything that raises blood sugars, because it is assumed that the glycemic spikes lead to increased fat accumulation, an increase in appetite and weight gain. This diet involves the consumption of complex and whole carbohydrates, as well as some types of fruit and vegetables.

Benefits. It can reduce the risk of diabetes and heart attack. In addition, it favors the consumption of foods that are part of each food group. You can eat as much as you want and when you like as long as the glycemic index is low.

Disadvantages. It is an illogical diet. For example, some types of fruit are fine, while others are not (as if that weren't enough, a ripe banana has a higher glycemic index than an unripe one). As a result, it can be a bit difficult to follow. Also, as the body's reactions to food change from day to day, it can be difficult to monitor its effectiveness.

Who should follow it? Opt for this diet if you are looking for a diet that allows you to lose weight slowly and progressively. Discard it if you want fast results and an easy-to-control diet.

Mediterranean diet

It focuses on the consumption of simple and fresh foods. It is based on the typical diet of Southern Italy and Greece, consisting of numerous varieties of fruit and vegetables, olive oil, non-GMO dairy products, dried fruit and little red meat. Those living in these regions have a lower risk of developing cardiovascular disease, cancer, diabetes and obesity.

Benefits. It does not openly rule out a particular food group, although it leaves little room for industrially processed junk foods. It includes complex carbohydrates, such as oats (great for most people), and occasionally a glass of red wine. It has been shown to be good for overall health and is fairly easy to follow, as long as the follower is aware of the decision made.

Disadvantages. Weight loss is not fast and the effects may be more internal than external. Since it is quite a varied diet, it is easy to assume that a food is fine, when it could be harmful. A handful of nuts is healthy, but a whole jar is not. Sometimes it is difficult to know when to contain portions.

Who should follow it? Try it if you intend to improve your overall health (rather than lose weight quickly) and you like the idea of avoiding processed foods, preferring fresh ones while following an intermittent fasting protocol. Forget if you want a quick loss of weight, don't know how to cook (few frozen foods are compatible with this diet) or have a limited budget.

Paleo diet

It is a recently developed diet that allows you to eat only the foods available in the time of primitive men, namely lean meats, fish, fruit, non-starchy vegetables, nuts and eggs. It totally excludes dairy products, processed foods and starchy vegetables, such as potatoes. It can significantly lower your blood sugar and, therefore, prove to be very healthy.

Benefits. It can promote strong weight loss, as long as it is followed correctly. It is based on the assumption of how humans should eat to get better. Also, don't count calories!

Disadvantages. You cannot eat potatoes and dairy products, because they are included in the list of prohibited foods even if they are generally considered healthy (like milk). Moreover, since some basic ingredients are excluded, it can be really difficult to eat out or have a particular dish prepared. In addition, there is the risk of overdoing it with some dish that is good for you, provided it is consumed in moderation.

Who should follow it? Choose this diet if you are an advocate of healthy eating and like to challenge yourself in the kitchen. Avoid it if you don't have the time and energy to try new cooking techniques or don't want to make a thousand changes to the restaurant menu. Also, it's not ideal for someone who can't live without dessert.

Asian diet

Known as the mother of all modern diets, the traditional Asian diet has a history of nearly 5,000 years and is now practiced by billions of people around the world. It focused on a natural, healthy and balanced diet based on fruit, vegetables and whole grains, with moderate consumption of eggs, lean meat and fish.

Those who follow it are also exposed to a lower risk of diabetes, high cholesterol, heart disease and stroke.

Benefits. It is completely natural, based on scientific research and 100% safe. It is balanced to meet all of your nutritional needs. No calculation is needed, but you can do it if you wish.

Disadvantages. You have to learn how to cook some Asian dishes, even if they are generally not complex. You have to give up almost all processed and junk foods.

Who should follow it? It is the perfect diet for those who want to eat healthily and cleanly, learn about other cultures and try new recipes in the kitchen.

Diet plans for weight loss

There is a plethora of diet programs, such as Weight Watchers, Jenny Craig and Nutrisystem, planned with menus, meetings and brochures to help you stay on track and motivated. Typically, they prescribe a low-calorie diet, but some also include low-fat foods.

Advantages. They are tailor-made for you. Some even provide for home delivery of what you need to eat. If you follow them carefully, it will be almost impossible to overshoot. In addition, you can count on a network of people ready to support you.

Disadvantages. In general, you only eat the foods included in the program, which by the way is paid for by the membership.

Who should follow it? Give it a try if you want to have something planned to help keep your life uncomplicated. It is also ideal for those women who need constant stimulation and find meetings and participation in support groups useful. However, if you like to cook and give space to creativity, this is not for you.

Cyclic diet

Recent studies are in favor of this type of diet which is divided as follows. Some days of the week are dedicated to the consumption of low-calorie foods, a couple of days are dedicated to a regular diet and only one to a high-calorie diet. This alternation prevents the body from getting used to the intermittent fasting protocol and therefore the metabolism remains active.

Advantages. There is no exclusion or limitation to any food group and there is a day in which you can "binge in a healthy way". You are not told when you can do it - you just have to organize yourself properly.

Disadvantages. You have to learn how to count calories, which can be a hassle especially in the beginning. You can't even give yourself too much freedom: just because you have a full calorie day, doesn't mean you can eat 30 cookies, otherwise you compromise the results.

Who should follow it? According to most of the research it appears that, when done correctly, it is quite healthy. If you want to see results, just make sure you consume lots of fruits, vegetables, lean meats and whole grains every day, regardless of the day. If you are a committed person and are interested in understanding how the body works, it could be for you. However, you also need to know your weaknesses. In fact, it's easy to give in to temptation, count calories and avoid losing sight of the ultimate goal.

The three-hour diet

You can eat every 3 hours to keep the metabolism active, otherwise the body will automatically run out of reserves. Eat light meals at regular times by adding a few 100-calorie snacks. However, you must avoid eating 3 hours before bedtime. If you want, you can consume precooked foods. As you can see, this goes against a standard intermittent fasting protocol as you can eat every three hours. We thought to include this diet in this list because it could be a viable option for some of you.

Benefits. You can eat everything, including less healthy dishes, as long as you can control the portions. It also helps you feel full because you eat all day and promotes a good balance between the various food groups.

Disadvantages. It could be easily mistaken. Freedom can lead you to go astray. Furthermore, there is not much scientific evidence to support the effectiveness of mini-meals.

Who should follow it? Try this diet if you feel like trying something different and are in the habit of snacking on a lot. Discard it if you want an effective method to help you lose weight fast or you don't have enough willpower to keep your commitment.

The new Beverly Hills diet

It is based on a very specific idea. In fact, for this diet it doesn't matter what you eat, but what counts is to do it at the right time and make the right food combinations. A correct combination of these two factors promotes digestion which prohibits the body to store fat. Supporters of this dietary regimen believe it is possible to lose 7 lbsin the initial phase which lasts 35 days.

Benefits. Believe it or not, there are no restrictions on calories or food groups. You don't have to calculate your calorie intake, but pay attention to when you eat. In addition to this, the consumption of fruits and vegetables is encouraged, which is good for the body.

Disadvantages. To begin with, there is no scientific evidence to support its effectiveness; in the beginning you can only eat fruit, which is not healthy at all. The rules are a bit confusing and difficult to follow (for example, once you have chosen a protein dish, you can only eat proteins; when you eat a certain type of fruit, then you have to move on to another and so on).

Who should follow it? Try this diet if you don't get along with portion control or food restrictions. If you're willing to splurge, you can buy books, DVDs, and meal plans. Avoid it if you are not committed and diligent.

Avoid crash diets

Crash diets are extreme diets that promise rapid weight loss, but the problem is that they rarely work. They often cause you to starve and, as a result, are bad for your health. When you want to lose weight, try to avoid the following types of diets.

- Purifying diets;
- Juice diets;
- Soup-based diets, such as cabbage or chicken
- Liquid based diets;
- The grapefruit diet.

Regardless of what kind of diet you decide to adopt, co-opt someone else's support if you can. This is especially important if you have chosen a difficult diet to follow. Knowing that you can count on someone is what you need to not lose heart.

This is why programs like Weight Watchers are enjoying some success. However, you don't need to subscribe to a certain program if you want support. In fact, you can just contact friends and family to have some form of support.

Combine diet and exercise

Each diet should be paired with physical activity, whether it's aerobics, weight lifting, or both. Whether you want to walk or run 3 miles, try to get moving. This way, the results will be really visible and it will be easier to continue the diet. Do at least 150 minutes of exercise a week to keep yourself healthy. If you want to lose weight, you should increase the training time to at least 5 hours.

Avoid motor activity only if you crack down on calorie restriction. Exercising continuously on an empty stomach carries health risks.

Whether you are on a diet or not, preferably choose organic and whole foods. The less they are processed, the more the nutrients they contain are preserved. This eating style can be expensive. To save money, buy in bulk or, if you can, shop at a fruit and vegetable store. Also, if you are lucky enough to have friends who are attentive to their nutrition, try to get organized with them to buy larger quantities at a better price.

Make sure your diet is flexible and enjoyable

You will not be able to follow it if it does not have these two characteristics:

- **Flexible**. There will be days when you want to go to a restaurant, days when you have nothing at home but pizza and days when you have no desire to respect your intermittent fasting protocol. A flexible diet that doesn't cause you to feel guilty when you go wrong is easier to implement in an intermittent fasting protocol.

- **Pleasant**. You don't have to be a scientist to understand that it's not the best to drink just water with a squeeze of lemon and maple juice for a week. If it were, it would be a recommended diet for everyone. Whatever type of diet you choose, make sure it allows you to eat foods you enjoy. Do you like meat? Try the Atkins diet. Do you love olive oil? Give the Mediterranean diet a try. The choices are not lacking and your intermittent fasting protocol can be adapted to different diets.

Ask your doctor for advice

The only person who knows your body almost as much as you do and who can give you a reliable opinion is your doctor. Therefore, you need to consult it before you seriously go on a diet. Every woman is different and some diets are not suitable for everyone.

This recommendation is especially true if you are pregnant, experiencing menopause, an elderly person, or if you have health problems. The last thing to hope for is that a new eating style will affect your health in a negative way. So, select a couple of diets that piqued your interest and talk to your doctor about them before implementing them in your intermittent fasting protocol.

Ask your doctor if they can recommend a dietician who will help you make a nutritional plan that fits your lifestyle and weight loss goal.

Chapter 20 - How to Follow an Intermittent Fasting Protocol During Menopause

When you reach the age of menopause it is normal for your body to change in many ways. This new condition can bring with it several symptoms, including fatigue and mood swings. Improving your intermittent fasting protocol can help mitigate negative effects and prevent health problems that can appear as you age. You should eat mostly healthy fruits, vegetables, proteins and fats. Foods rich in nutrients, such as calcium, are useful for controlling the symptoms of menopause. Learn to avoid foods that are bad for you, such as those that are high in sugar or high in fat, to keep you fit and healthy even as you age.

Choose starches that are good for your health

Starches should be the staple of your intermittent fasting protocol when you enter menopause. Choosing the right type makes a noticeable difference. Choose starches in natural foods, such as potatoes, to keep your body strong during the menopause.

Regular potatoes, but also sweet potatoes, are an excellent source of starch when cooked healthily. Give up the habit of peeling them and cook them in the oven or steam rather than frying them. From now on you should only eat whole foods. When shopping at the grocery store, avoid refined rice, pasta and bread and opt for the wholemeal version.

Remember that starches need to be at the core of your daily diet, but you also need to make sure you don't overdo portions. Approximately one third of the food eaten in a day must consist of starches.

Eat five servings of fruit and vegetables a day even when following an intermittent fasting protocol

From an early age you will have heard that fruit and vegetables are important and as age advances they become more and more fundamental. If you want to be healthy during menopause, make sure you eat at least five servings of fresh fruit and vegetables every day, even if you are following an intermittent fasting protocol. In fact, at this point of your life it is much more important to be healthy than sticking to a specific intermittent fasting protocol.

You can eat fruit when you feel like having a snack between meals. An apple, half a banana or a peach counts as one serving. Try to eat some vegetables with each meal. When it's time to choose your lunch side dish, opt for a salad instead of fries. In the evening, prepare steamed vegetables to combine with starches and proteins.

Choose the right proteins

As we have seen in a previous chapter, as we age, the daily requirement for protein increases. To keep yourself healthy and avoid getting too many calories while eating more protein foods, it's important to select them appropriately. Lean meats, dairy products, fish and eggs should be a regular part of your intermittent fasting protocol.

You should eat fish at least twice a week. Buy fresh fish instead of smoked or preserved fish which normally contain a lot of salt. Choose the leanest varieties of meat. Chicken meat (skin removed) is a good choice.

If you are a vegetarian, eggs can be a good source of protein. Legumes, nuts, and oil seeds are other healthy options.

Generally speaking, when we talk about a healthy intermittent fasting protocol, we think we have to completely eliminate fats, but in truth some types of fats are necessary to keep the body healthy. To stay healthy, you have to opt for those contained in natural foods, for example in extra virgin olive oil, dried fruit, oil seeds and avocados. Instead, avoid foods that are high in saturated or trans fat.

Soy and its derivatives can help you with hormonal problems

If you are experiencing symptoms, for example you have mood swings, eating soy and its derivatives can positively affect the delicate balance of your hormonal system.
Try substituting tofu for meat a couple of times a week. Replace cow's milk with soy milk from time to time for breakfast. When you go to the baker, also buy some soy rolls in addition to the wholemeal one.

Take zinc and iron to keep your immune system strong

They are both very useful for increasing the body's defenses during menopause. By having a strong immune system, you won't risk getting sick easily. Try to eat foods rich in zinc and iron at this time in your life.

Many animal-based foods contain zinc, such as fish, seafood, and calf's liver. Plant-based options include oilseeds, nuts, and whole grains. To get the iron you need, you can eat beef, pork or lamb, fish, and seafood. Plant-based options include spinach, mustard leaves, kale, parsley, and cauliflower.

Improve your mood with a healthy intermittent fasting protocol

Mood swings are a common symptom during menopause. Fortunately, there are many foods that promote a good mood in a natural way. The amino acid tryptophan can induce a sense of serenity and contentment.

Cottage cheese is high in tryptophan and generally healthy. You can eat it for breakfast with fruit if you are feeling down in terms of mood. Tryptophan is also contained in oats, so you can start the day right with a cup of oat flakes too.

Turkey is another good source of tryptophan. If the moodiness shows up in the middle of the day, you can eat it in a sandwich.

In addition to eating foods that are rich in tryptophan, be careful not to skip breakfast. Otherwise you will cause negative effects on health, metabolism and feel bad mood. If you are following an intermittent fasting protocol, we advise you to eat breakfast and then have the fasting period. In fact, you need to eat something as soon as you wake up if you want to be full of energy and fight bad moods.

During menopause, the body's bone structure may weaken. By increasing your calcium consumption you can counteract this process. Nonetheless, it is important to get calcium from the right foods to keep the whole body healthy.

Milk and other dairy products, such as yogurt, contain both the calcium and the protein you need during menopause. It's best to choose skim milk and low-fat cheeses to fill up on calcium without getting too much fat.

Stay away from fast food and all junk food in general. All those products are full of salt and sugar. During menopause, people tend to gain weight easily because metabolism slows down, so it is best to completely avoid high-calorie and unhealthy foods. Do your best to avoid fast food, fried foods, and sweets. You can indulge in a dessert once or twice a week and not as a daily habit.

Stop drinking sweetened drinks. Sweetened drinks have been found to interfere with the body's ability to absorb calcium, so you should avoid them, especially with meals. Still water is the best choice for staying healthy while following an intermittent fasting protocol. If you feel the need to add some flavor to the water, you can flavor it with pieces of fresh fruit.

Keep portions under control

Use small plates and glasses. When eating out, try to eat only part of what's on your plate and have the rest packaged to bring it home. The larger the portions, the greater the amount of calories, fat and sugar, so you should try to limit your serving whenever possible.

Since your metabolism is slowing down, you inevitably need to consume fewer calories than ever before. Furthermore, as we age we tend to do less and less movement. For these reasons, portions that were once acceptable may now be too large for your calorie requirement. You should calculate how many calories your body needs to receive each day based on your age and level of physical activity and talk to your doctor or nutritionist to know how to properly modify your diet and stay within limits.

It can be useful to understand what quantity a portion visually corresponds to in order to be able to calculate the correct doses by eye when eating out or while cooking. For example, a portion of meat or fish weighs about a pound and is about the size of a deck of cards. For example, a serving of almond cream is about the size of a ping-pong ball or two full tablespoons (30 g). One serving of cereal would fill a cupcake case.

Cut down on your sugar intake. In addition to making you fat it can cause several age-related health problems. During menopause, you should do your best to get as little as possible.

Any drink you drink should be sugar-free. Ideal choices include water (plain or flavored for example with lemon, mint or berries), unsweetened tea and herbal teas. Please, make sure you don't sweeten your breakfast cereals. You can satisfy your craving for sweet foods with ingredients like vanilla, almonds, ripe fruit, dates, dried figs, raisins and cinnamon.

Chapter 21 - How to Follow an Intermittent Fasting Protocol During Menopause: Part 2

During the third age and around menopause, many women have problems with being overweight. In this stage of life the weight gain is partly due to hormonal reasons, as the changes that occur in the body predispose to the accumulation of fat in the central area of the body. However, hormones are not the only ones responsible, and during menopause, gaining weight is by no means inevitable. This phenomenon is also often related to factors such as aging, lifestyle and genetics. If you feel frustrated by putting on a few pounds, you need to know that you are not alone and that there is no need to despair. It is possible to intervene to reverse the course by exercising, following a healthy intermittent fasting protocol and leading a healthy lifestyle.

Rule out any underlying conditions

Gaining weight during menopause is usually due to a natural aging process. However, you should still make sure that the phenomenon is not caused by a potentially serious underlying condition. Contact your doctor to rule out any diseases that may be responsible for weight gain.

For example, your doctor may need to determine if you have hypothyroidism, a disorder that tends to affect many women over the years. The thyroid plays a vital role in regulating metabolism. If it does insufficient work, the metabolism will slow down, causing weight gain.

Weight gain can also be related to conditions such as diabetes (as a side effect of insulin), water retention, use of corticosteroids, Cushing's syndrome or vitamin D deficiency. It is better to consult a doctor to rule out these possibilities.

Muscle mass decreases over the years, as a result it becomes increasingly difficult to manage your weight. Doing weight lifting helps to develop muscles again and lower the risk of osteoporosis. Do strength exercises that target major muscle groups at least twice a week. For starters, do cardio and weightlifting exercises every other day. As you gain strength, try combining the two workouts for maximum results.

To develop muscle mass you need to do exercises that involve the use of weights and that test the muscles through resistance work. For example, consider lifting weights, using resistance bands, bodyweight exercises (such as pushups) and others. If you're gardening, digging and shoveling are also effective moves for good strength training.

Menopausal women should avoid sit-ups, as they stress the spine. Try exercises like the plank, while for the lower body you can opt for movements like lunges and squats.

Strength training also has another benefit: it protects the bones. The 5 years following the onset of menopause are often risky, as bone loss tends to occur quite quickly at this stage. Weight lifting helps maintain good bone density and it works wonderfully with an intermittent fasting protocol.

Add cardiovascular conditioning

Aerobic activity (often also called cardiovascular activity) is another important factor in maintaining a dynamic lifestyle, allowing you to burn fat and speed up your metabolism. It also helps lower blood pressure, improve lipid profile, reduce insulin sensitivity and even decrease the risk of heart disease or type 2 diabetes.

To begin with, train for 30 minutes a day, three times a week. Take a brisk walk on the treadmill or jog at a brisk pace. For a varied workout that doesn't stress your knees, use the elliptical. Aim for a total of 150 minutes of moderate physical activity or 75 minutes of strenuous physical activity per week.

Also, choose exercises that you like. For example, you can go hiking, cycling, playing golf or dancing. Physical activity should be done primarily for health reasons, but that doesn't mean it can't be fun.

Seek support

Strictly following a training plan is not always easy. Sometimes it is useful to know that you can count on friends or relatives who help you keep motivation high, to be responsible and to follow a dynamic intermittent fasting protocol. If you're having a hard time staying consistent, look for tricks to keep you on track. For example, invite a friend to exercise with you or sign up for a class.

There are numerous opportunities to play sports with other people. For example, you could join a running group or team. You could also sign up for a class at the gym, where you will be in the company of people with similar goals to yours.

If you are a tech enthusiast, try using an app or watching training videos. There are numerous apps to try, such as Hot5, RunKeeper or GymPact. The latter, for example, leads to a commitment to train a certain number of times each week, with penalties for failure and rewards for success.

Choose activities that are right for you. It is important to consider your interests and tastes, whether it be aerobics, climbing or roller derby.

Calculate your calorie needs

Weight is closely related to the amount of calories that are consumed and disposed of. In general, an adult woman over 50 needs 1600-2000 calories per day. However, the exact figures depend on variables such as age, type of physical activity performed, and more.

To know your needs, you can first calculate your basal metabolic rate or MB, which indicates the energy expenditure to perform vital metabolic functions. For women, the equation is usually as follows: 655.1 + (19,2 * weight [lbs]) + (1.8 * height [cm]) - (4.7 * age [years]).

Now, change this number by considering the type of physical activity you do. Multiply the MB by one of the following numbers: 1.2 for a sedentary lifestyle, 1.375 for a slightly active lifestyle, 1.55 for a moderately active lifestyle, 1.725 for a very active lifestyle, and 1.9 for a lifestyle particularly active.

For example, imagine you are a 55-year-old woman with a height of 167cm and a weight of 130lbs. Your MB is approximately 1322. Being moderately active, multiply 1322 by 1.55 and you will get 2050. This is your daily calorie requirement, which allows you to maintain your healthy weight.

It takes about 3500 calories a week to lose half a pound. Once you've calculated your calorie needs, you can try to achieve this by counting calories or keeping a food diary. Just make sure you do it correctly. Don't consume fewer calories than your MB indicates, and never consume less than 1200 calories per day. In fact, it is best to consult a nutritionist to ensure that you are safely losing weight.

Generally speaking, processed and refined foods are less healthy. They generally contain fewer nutrients (vitamins and minerals), more fat, more additives and more sodium. Better to avoid these types of products and replace them with whole grains, fruits and vegetables.

Here are some examples of processed foods: refined grains, simple carbohydrates, such as white bread and rice, products containing refined flours. Also avoid junk food, fast food, and foods containing trans fat or corn syrup.

Try to replace refined foods with their healthy alternatives. Replace classic breakfast cereals with a bowl of oatmeal made with whole grain oatmeal. Replace white rice with brown rice, pearl barley, or quinoa. You can also make a large baked potato, but avoid using too much butter or fatty spreads to make it healthier.

Eat more fruits and vegetables

In addition to being rich in nutrients, they help you feel full. They are essential for a healthy diet and often contain fewer calories than other foods. To sweeten oatmeal and get potassium, garnish it with a sliced banana. If you're craving sweets, snack on grapes or berries. Prefer pumpkin noodles and make a mushroom-based sauce instead of meat. Use garlic and onion in cooking to prevent inflammation.

Fill up on dark leafy greens, like kale. They are an excellent source of calcium, which is particularly important during and after menopause for strong bones. Use them to fill sandwiches or make salads, or sauté them with garlic and olive oil to make a tasty side dish.

It is important to avoid getting too many calories in the form of liquids. Alcoholic beverages are high-calorie. If your family has had several cases of heart disease, you can indulge in a glass of red wine a day, but don't go any further. Avoid spirits, beer, and drinks containing added sugar.

Don't be afraid to eat fat

Many women believe they are harmful or make you fat, but that's not entirely true. Lipids not only play a vital role in following a healthy intermittent fasting protocol, they also contain more calories than carbohydrates and proteins.

Consequently, foods that are naturally high in fat have a high satiating power. In fact, according to some studies, high-fat diets can lead to more weight loss than low-fat intermittent fasting protocols.

Many doctors thought that eating a diet high in saturated fat increases the risk of heart disease. Apparently this is also not true: as long as you incorporate them correctly and in moderation, products like butter, coconut oil, and red meat may not be as harmful as you thought.

While it is possible to eat saturated fats, you should still avoid trans fats. By being chemically modified to have longer storage times, they can affect the risk of contracting heart disease, as well as cause insulin resistance and inflammation.

Hormone replacement therapy (HRT)

In addition to increasing estrogen and progesterone levels, which are decreasing, it can help you lose weight or maintain a healthy weight. However, it is a personal decision that must be made together with your gynecologist.

When combined with exercise, HRT helps you stay fit and protect your bones. However, it can also pose risks for some women. Be sure to discuss this with your doctor, who is aware of your medical history and the consequences you may face.

Consider bioidentical hormone replacement therapy (BHRT) instead of traditional HRT. This treatment mimics the functions of human hormones, while HRT uses synthetic hormones derived from horse urine. BHRT was associated with fewer side effects.

Clean the house using ecological products

Pesticides, pollutants and chemicals found in detergents can increase the risk of hormone imbalances and gaining weight. Look for eco-friendly products made from organic or all-natural ingredients. Better yet, clean up using natural products you already have at home - baking soda, white vinegar, and fresh lemon juice are just as effective and leave no chemical residue.

Chapter 22 - How to Improve Food Digestion in an Intermittent Fasting Protocol

In this chapter we are going to discuss the importance of having a fast and healthy food digestion process when following an intermittent fasting protocol. We will also share some tips on how to improve your digestion after turning 50.

The digestive process breaks down food into small parts to allow the body to benefit from the energy and nutrients it contains. Different foods are broken down in different ways, some more quickly than others. Although the duration of digestion is mainly due to the natural mechanisms of the human body, there are some things you can do to digest better and faster. Read on to learn how to digest food quickly.

Exercise regularly

An increase in physical activity helps keep food moving in the digestive system. As a result, the speed and quality of digestion can improve. Exercising helps you prevent constipation. Furthermore, it accelerates digestion as it reduces the time that food spends in the large intestine, thus also limiting the amount of water that the body reabsorbs from the stool. Movement also promotes natural smooth muscle contractions in the digestive tract, accelerating the breakdown of food. However, after eating, it is best to wait about an hour before exercising so that the blood has a chance to concentrate in the digestive tract rather than having to replenish the heart and other working muscles.

When you sleep, the organs of the digestive system have time to recover, which increases their ability to digest food quickly and efficiently. Improving your sleep pattern can have far-reaching digestive benefits.

Do not go to sleep immediately after eating; wait two or three hours so that the body has time to digest. Try sleeping on your left side. In fact, studies have shown that sleeping on the left side of the body increases digestive capacity.

Drink lots of fluids

Taking liquids during or after meals, especially water and herbal teas, promotes good digestion. Water helps the body break down food, while also allowing it to stay properly hydrated. Proper hydration of the body allows you to produce the right amount of saliva and fluids in the stomach. Water also keeps the stool soft, preventing constipation. Last but not least, water is crucial for the body's proper use of fiber, essential components for digestion.

Eat high-fiber foods

High-fiber foods promote digestion in several ways. These foods can help speed up the process, reducing constipation and keeping the intestines healthy.

The fibers work by absorbing water and adding weight and volume to the stool. For this to happen it is necessary to take an adequate amount of water, otherwise you could suffer from constipation. By giving more volume to the stool, foods rich in fiber regulate digestion. They can also help reduce gas, bloating and alleviate episodes of dysentery.

Foods rich in fiber include the following:
- wholemeal flour products

- vegetables
- fruits
- legumes
- nuts and seeds.

Yogurt is an excellent natural source of probiotics and other live cultures, essential for proper digestion. The benefits of yogurt on digestion are believed to come from the fact that it stimulates the growth of good bacteria thanks to the live cultures it naturally contains. Furthermore, it reduces the time it takes to heal from infections and also decreases the immune system response in individuals with irritable bowel syndrome.

It also reduces the time it takes food to travel through the intestinal tract. As you can see, yogurt is not only delicious, but it also helps your gut in many different ways.

The secret power of ginger

For thousands of years, ginger has been used as a digestive remedy and its popularity has continued to the present day. Ginger is known for its ability to stimulate the release of enzymes in the digestive tract, thereby increasing its effectiveness and promoting good digestion.

Ginger has been shown to increase the contractions of the stomach muscles, helping to move food faster to the upper part of the small intestine.

Prefer low-fat foods, avoiding fatty or fried ones. High-fat foods, as well as fried foods, can cause heartburn and acid reflux, as they destroy the stomach's ability to properly break down the contents. These foods are difficult for your stomach to digest, so they slow down the whole process.

Some examples of deep-fried or high-fat foods are sausages, french fries, ice cream, butter, and cheese.

Avoid very spicy foods, preferring delicate ones. Spicy foods can irritate the throat and esophagus, causing heartburn and acid reflux. In addition, these foods can damage the gastrointestinal tract, slowing digestion and causing episodes of dysentery and other digestive disorders.

Limit or avoid dairy products and red meat

As a rule, yogurt is beneficial for almost all people, however, if you have symptoms of lactose intolerance, it should be avoided just like all other dairy products. Although the exact mechanism by which dairy products cause constipation and indigestion is not yet known, it has been proven that they can hinder the digestive process. Lactose intolerance can cause abdominal bloating, gas formation and indigestion, and disorders that can be the result of poor or slowed digestion.

Red meat can cause constipation, hindering the regular evacuation of stool, a necessary condition for rapid digestion. There are many reasons why red meat negatively affects digestion. Among them, the main ones are the following.

- It is high in fat, so the body needs more time to process it.
- It is rich in iron, another possible cause of constipation.

Prefer natural foods to processed ones. Foods that have undergone intense industrial processing are more difficult to digest; therefore prefer natural ones, which do not contain high doses of preservatives, additives and other harmful chemicals. Eat whole fruits, vegetables, rice and pasta, legumes, nuts, seeds and other natural foods to aid the digestive process, also making it more efficient.

Chew each bite carefully. Even if it is too often underestimated, chewing kicks off the digestive process. When you chew properly you increase the surface area of the food particles, allowing greater access by enzymes. Exposing a large surface area of food to saliva is a great way to initiate easy and efficient digestion.

Probiotic supplements

Probiotics are bacteria capable of promoting the natural balance of intestinal microorganisms. Some medical studies have indicated that, when taken as supplements, they can facilitate digestion by increasing the amount of beneficial bacteria found in the gut. Probiotics are also contained in many varieties of foods, so if you don't intend to take them through a supplement, you can include them in your diet to reap the multiple benefits.

As the food supplement market is subject to little regulation, special care should be taken when choosing probiotics. Read the product label carefully, making sure it contains the following information.

- Genus, species and strain of the probiotic (such as Lactobacillus rhamnosus GG);
- Number of organisms that will be alive by the expiration date;
- Doses;
- Name and contacts of the manufacturing company.

It is very important to know the types of probiotic strains contained in the selected supplement as each individual tends to react better to some than others. The best thing to do is to choose a product that contains several different probiotic strains.

Digestive enzyme supplement

This is an over-the-counter product that can help facilitate digestion by providing the body with an addition of natural enzymes. The job of enzymes is to break down food into its different components, allowing the body to absorb it more easily. When these enzymes work effectively they make digestion fast and efficient.

Digestive enzymes are produced by four glands in the human body, but mainly by the pancreas.

While some practitioners of alternative medicine deny the claimed benefits of natural supplement manufacturers, most mainstream doctors argue that more in-depth studies are needed to determine the true effects of enzyme supplements. Among the best-selling digestive enzyme supplements we find the following ones.

- Zimase. It naturally contains digestive enzymes, useful for optimizing the enzymatic functions of the entire digestive tract and promoting the physiological digestive process.

- Prolife 10. Contains 10 strains of lactic ferments selected from those with the highest probiotic value; these characteristics make it useful for rebalancing the alterations of the intestinal bacterial flora.

- Similase Total. It promotes the physiological digestion of lactose, complex sugars, vegetable fibers, fats and proteins.

By following these advice you can make sure to have a functional digestive system that will allow you to improve the quality of your intermittent fasting protocol. Please, after you reach the age of 50, do not underestimate the power of having an effective digestive system, as it can truly make or break your ability to lose weight and burn fat. In fact, research has shown that even if following an intermittent fasting protocol, women over 50 tend to struggle to lose weight when they have digestive problems.

Chapter 23 - How to Naturally Improve Metabolism During Intermittent Fasting

As we have seen in previous chapters as well, having a fast metabolism can improve your chances of losing weight while following an intermittent fasting protocol. In the next few pages we are going to discuss the strategies you can implement to boost your metabolism while following an intermittent fasting protocol.

Metabolism is a biological process that occurs within the body and which determines how quickly the body transforms calories into energy. Those with a fast metabolism burn fat first, while those with a slow metabolism do not. Some women believe that having a fast metabolism results in greater weight loss and that having a high body mass index (BMI) is indicative of a slow metabolism. Although these ideas are generally wrong, changing the basal metabolic rate (MB, or the energy expenditure of an organism at rest) allows you to lose a small amount of fat more quickly without doing anything. The metabolism is mainly regulated by factors such as genetics, age and sex, but it is possible to intervene to positively affect its functioning in a completely natural way.

Avoid foods of industrial origin

The processed foods are those full of salt, sugar and fat, completely devoid (or almost) of nutrients and vitamins. Sure, they're delicious, but they slow down your metabolism. As if this were not enough, they do not satiate and are addictive, causing you to put on weight. Therefore, we suggest you avoid candy, fizzy drinks, potato chips, candy, fast food, and other processed foods.

You can indulge in a treat from time to time, just make sure it's healthy, natural and organic. For example, you can learn to make cookies, muffins, and other desserts at home.

Junk and processed food slows down the metabolic rate, while healthy food speeds it up. Fruits and vegetables are at the top of the list of foods that naturally stimulate metabolism. Almost any type of fruit or vegetable will do. Add more leafy greens, such as spinach, lettuce, and kale. Tasty fruits like apples, strawberries and pineapples are also recommended. If you don't like eating salads and fruit, try browning or baking asparagus or eggplant. If you're constantly in a hurry, try investing in a good blender for making fruit and vegetable-based drinks.

Season with spices. Spicy foods can temporarily speed up metabolism by about 8% above a woman's normal rate. Additionally, a spicy dish promotes a longer-lasting sense of satiety than one that isn't. Sprinkle cayenne pepper on the potatoes or season the sandwiches with sriracha sauce. Ground red pepper is great for adding pungent notes to pizza or pasta. Chili is a spicy dish perfect for warming up on colder days. Try dressing kale, broccoli, and other vegetables with some hot sauce. Incorporate sauces and spicy additives in moderation. Overdoing it can cause ulcers and heartburn.

Proteins and metabolism

Lean proteins, such as chicken breast, tofu, nuts and legumes, can speed up your metabolism. Proteins are more difficult to digest than fats, salts and sugars, so they require a more demanding assimilation process. This leads to a greater expenditure of energy which stimulates the metabolism. If you like chicken or turkey, cook it in the oven or grill. Fried meat, like fried chicken, will only add empty calories to your diet. Avoid processed meats, such as hot dogs, bacon, salami, beef sausages, and fast food burgers. Consumption of these foods has been linked to cancer and heart disease. Do not eat cheeses or other processed milk products, including those containing large amounts of salt or emulsifiers. For example, you should avoid cheese sauces, such as the one for nachos.

Water, green tea and coffee

Water plays a very important role in every single cellular process in the body. Since dehydration is essential for turning fat into energy, it can slow down your metabolism.

The amount of water you need to drink every day depends on your body. Try to consume half your body weight (in pounds) in fluid ounces. You can do this calculation on any search engine. For example, if you weigh 120 pounds, you should drink 60 fluid ounces (about 1.8 liters) per day.

If you don't like still water, try flavored water. It is available in many stores, but it can also be flavored at home by placing lemon or cucumber slices in a jug and letting them rest for a few hours. Bring a bottle of water wherever you go and drink regularly.

Green tea is a rich source of antioxidants called catechins and plays a vital role in stimulating the metabolism. Unsweetened green tea increases the calorie burn rate. In addition, it reduces cholesterol, fights cardiovascular disease, prevents cancer and Alzheimer's. Use it as a substitute for sugary sodas and fruit juices.

Caffeine can speed up your metabolism at a rate of between 5 and 8%. While it doesn't raise your basal metabolic rate as effectively as water or green tea, incorporating a cup of coffee with breakfast or after lunch can help. Limit yourself to just 2 or 3 cups a day, so you don't risk a caffeine overdose.

Weight lifting and HIIT

Cardiovascular and resistance exercises play a very important role in any training program, but weight lifting is much more effective in speeding up the metabolism. Try bicep curls, barbell squats, and bench presses to strengthen yourself and increase your basal metabolic rate.

To understand how much weight you should be lifting, start with less weight and gradually increase it. Before you begin to feel intense effort, you should be able to do 14 or 22 repetitions of an exercise.

For example, if you do 20 bicep curls using a certain weight and feel your muscles "burn", then the weight is ideal. If you can do them without feeling any discomfort, add 2 lbs and try to do another set.

Do not lift excessive loads. If the exertion is particularly intense, or your arms are shaking while lifting, take a break and try a short session of cardiovascular exercises. You may also be able to reduce the weight you lift or do fewer reps. Lifting excessive loads can cause injury.

Intensive sessions can cause the body to burn calories even after a workout. High Intensity Interval Workouts (HIIT) are effective in benefiting from the so-called afterburn effect. As the name suggests, high-intensity interval workouts include short but intense exercise intervals alternating with intervals of inactivity or characterized by less intense exercise. HIIT workouts include many types of exercises, including weight lifting, running, and bodyweight movements.

If you are a beginner, proceed step by step. For example, try to sprint at full speed for 20 seconds. As you build up and improve your endurance, try sprinting for 30 seconds, then 40, and so on.

When you train with the HIIT methodology, use a stopwatch. For example, if you want to do 20 bicep curls in 30 seconds, set your stopwatch for 30 seconds, then start doing the exercise. Don't sacrifice proper execution for speed. Always maintain proper posture, especially when lifting weights. Always warm up for about 10 minutes before you start exercising.

Take short intervals. It is impossible and even dangerous to train at maximum intensity for long periods of time. Each interval should not exceed 60 seconds.

Physical activity and physical exertion in general can improve basal metabolic rate. Simple activities like getting up and walking around talking on the phone, taking the stairs instead of taking the elevator, moving around while sitting at your desk in the office, and so on can burn even more calories.

Get used to taking short walks around the house or workplace, riding a bicycle instead of in the car, doing push-ups and sit-ups at the end of the day. Remember that even the simplest activities stimulate your metabolism and help burn fat effectively.

Metabolism, sleep and stress

If you deprive yourself of sleep, you risk slowing your metabolism. Adults should sleep at least 7 hours per night. If you don't get enough sleep, do something to increase your rest hours. Try to go to sleep and wake up at the same time every time. Use an alarm to keep track of times. Make the bedroom dark, quiet, and cool.

Do not use the bed or bedroom for activities other than rest. For example, don't read, watch television, or play video games. Avoid eating large meals before bed. You shouldn't eat 2 or 3 hours before bedtime.

If you feel tense and find it difficult to relax, try to manage your stress in a healthy way. Yoga, deep breathing, and regular exercise are all proven methods of reducing stress. Everyone responds differently to various anti-stress techniques. Experiment with various methods to find one that suits your needs.

If you have a particularly demanding or stressful job, look for a job that works best for you and don't overload yourself with too many optional extra projects. Getting enough sleep helps fight stress. Try to get at least 7 hours of sleep a night. If you suffer from severe anxiety or chronic stress, try seeing a therapist.

These specialists are tasked with helping people identify effective ways to relieve anxiety and stress.

Replace negative thoughts with thoughts that make you feel good. For example, if you get stressed out by thoughts like "I'm going to be bad at work", close your eyes and imagine that thought is a red balloon. Visualize yourself letting it go and see it fly away. Then, imagine being overwhelmed by millions of blue balloons, each with a positive thought, such as "Today is going to be a great day" or "I am proud of what I have achieved".
Whatever you do to improve your thoughts, please don't drink or use drugs to combat stress.

Prefer cool temperatures

Cold tends to increase metabolism. In the winter months, resist the temptation to set the radiators to maximum. Keeping the temperature at 18° C will not only allow you to save on your bill, it will also stimulate the basal metabolism. When it's hot, cool off by sipping iced drinks and keeping the air conditioning on. If you don't have air conditioning, turn on the fan.

Alternatively, when it's hot, go to a friend's house that has air conditioning, or go to a public place like a coffee shop or mall.

Chapter 24 - How to Eat Healthy When Your Have Little Time

Something that all women over 50 have in common is the fact that time is always an issue for them. In fact, nowadays life tends to be quite busy and it is normal to have issues regarding the preparation of meals for an intermittent fasting protocol. This is why we have decided to dedicate a chapter of this book to a few tips that can help you deal with this problem. We hope you can find some valuable tips to maximize your time while preparing the meals for your intermittent fasting protocol.

The busy schedule often makes it difficult to follow a healthy intermittent fasting protocol. You may not have time to go to the grocery store and prepare home cooked meals every night. The solution is to prepare dishes in advance for those times when you are in a hurry, so that you are guaranteed healthy meals and snacks that are readily available and that you are not tempted to eat unhealthy. By making certain changes in your daily routine and following a few tips, you will be able to eat properly while having a busy life.

Read the entire restaurant menu

Even if you have the best of intentions, sometimes you may have no alternatives and be forced to eat at fast food restaurants or get ready-made meals at the supermarket. However, it's a good idea to read the entire menu or go through the self-service to learn about the healthiest options available.

Look at the menu on the restaurant's website before choosing dishes and make sure there is some healthy solution. Alternatively, learn the menu of your favorite diner by heart. Identify a few dishes that fit into your healthy diet plan and stick to those.

Check the nutritional values of the various dishes. Restaurant chains that have more than 20 locations must report the nutritional information of the different dishes on the website and within the restaurant itself. Find dishes that meet your calorie needs and other nutrition guidelines.

Don't eat combination dishes. They are the ones with the highest caloric value you find in fast food restaurants. Just grab a sandwich or roll if possible.

Avoid heavily fried foods as much as possible. Most fast food chains also offer grilled versions of the different sandwiches, wraps or other dishes. Choose dishes cooked on the grill rather than fried, to reduce the amount of fat.

Remember that fast food isn't the only solution you have for a quick meal. Many places serve soups, salads, low-calorie sandwiches, as well as other not too elaborate, low-calorie dishes that are slightly healthier.

Use the smartphone app of your local map or do a quick online search to find alternative venues nearby. Look for something other than the usual fast food or rotisserie.

Remember that even though some restaurants offer fresh salads and sandwiches, these foods are not always low-calorie. Also, as already mentioned, don't forget to read the menu and the nutritional content of the dishes on the web page before going to the restaurant.

Stop at a supermarket for a quick meal

If you're hungry and don't have the time to cook, go to a grocery store for some quick, healthy dishes. Most well-stocked supermarkets offer several options that fit well into your busy lifestyle.

If you don't have time at all, grab something from the salads or hot dishes department. Choose lean proteins, vegetables, fruits, and whole grains. Avoid dishes that are particularly high in fat (such as frozen cheese pasta) or fried foods (such as chicken).

Many supermarkets also sell pre-prepared dishes and pre-packaged cold salads (such as chicken or tuna). Watch out for calorie and fat content, but a small serving of chicken salad and a piece of fruit make for a great quick meal.

Not all dishes need to be completely cooked at home from scratch. Some of the supermarkets offer relatively healthy, as well as quick, solutions. Surprisingly, even at gas stations with a grocery store you will sometimes find healthier dishes than fast food.

The healthy meals you can find at the convenience store are low-calorie frozen meals (but pay attention to the sodium content), low-calorie canned soups (but always check the amount of sodium present), single portions of dried fruit or food protein (many stores sell small packs of lean protein, such as nuts, cheese, hard-boiled or sliced eggs, accompanied by a fruit or vegetable).

The foods that you must avoid are those with high calories (such as very stuffed pizza or chicken nuggets), fried foods that you find in the rotisserie department, canned pasta, processed meat (such as hot dogs) and sandwiches or rolls of industrial production.

Eat the dishes you find in stores with awareness and moderation. Sometimes what makes this food "comfortable" is its excessive processing. This aspect does not always affect the nutritional value, but in other cases it can compromise the quality of the food. Always be very cautious and use common sense.

Prepare the fruit and vegetables in advance

Washing, cutting and cooking fruit and vegetables is typically the longest and most tedious part of preparing meals. Reduce cooking times by anticipating this job.

If you can, start preparing your fruit and vegetables as soon as you get home after purchasing them. Keep them on the kitchen counter and try to get rid of this chore as soon as possible.

Wash them thoroughly, dry them and store them in suitable containers or in the refrigerator. If you plan to eat them raw, you don't have to do anything else.

If you want to cook vegetables, cut or mince them and place them in sealable plastic bags. When you want to cook them, all you have to do is put them in the pot and cook them! Consider using a food processor to quickly chop fruit and vegetables. If you decide to use them as a side dish for lunch or snacks, divide them into the right portions already and keep them until you are ready to consume them.

Prepare full meals in advance

If your meals are already cooked and ready, it becomes much easier to eat right, despite a busy life. The key to success is preparation; in this way it is easier to make healthier food choices. You don't have to eat ready-made meals all the time, but they are the perfect solution on certain occasions.

Prepare breakfasts to eat on the go. Some meals and foods are easy to eat even while you are driving or traveling by train to work. Have foods like these on hand: cereal or protein bars, ready-made smoothies or hard-boiled eggs.

You can also prepare your meals during the weekend. For example, cook some scrambled eggs, get some cheese or scones and place them in the refrigerator well packaged. All you have to do is take them and heat them in the microwave when you want to eat them.

You can also organize lunches and dinners in advance. Make salads with lettuce, vegetables, lean proteins, any ingredients you like and store them in airtight containers. When you want to eat them you will only have to season them. Stews and other types of dishes can also be cooked completely in advance and reheated when you need them.

Get a slow cooker

The slow cooker is the best friend of those with a busy life. It allows you to cook the dish throughout the day and you can enjoy a hot, simple and ready dish as soon as you return home in the evening.

Some models are relatively cheap and can have different prices, ranging from 20 to 200 dollars. Choose a pot with the size, shape and characteristics that suit your needs.

The slow cooker is also great for preparing large portions. This way you'll have leftovers to reuse, extra meals or portions to freeze and enjoy later.

Prepare more of the same dish

If you have an evening or two in which you can indulge in cooking, consider doubling the amount of the dishes you prepare. It can be useful to have some leftovers for lunches or dinners for the following days. This way, you no longer have to worry about going to the supermarket or cooking again, as the meal is ready.

If you don't like the idea of eating leftovers or prefer to eat something different, just double down on part of the recipe. For example, if you are cooking chicken rolls, you can grill extra meat (with or without seasonings) to use in other combinations (such as grilled chicken with Caesar salad or chicken with broccoli and brown rice).

It's a good idea to cook larger quantities even if you don't need any leftovers for the foreseeable future. You can always divide them into single portions and freeze them for the days when you are in a hurry. You will be happy to have your meal ready, which just needs to be reheated.

Never run out of healthy snacks

It is worth having snacks or other convenient, ready-to-eat foods to eat when you feel the need and are particularly busy. By doing so, you will not be tempted to eat junk food.

Take some time each week to prepare healthy snacks. Divide them into individual portions and refrigerate them until you want to eat them.

Here are some healthy snack ideas. Carrots and hummus, apple and cheese sticks, celery and peanut butter, or a Greek yogurt with fruit.

You will be less inclined to give in to the temptation to eat something sweet and unhealthy by having these snacks ready and readily available.

Decide the meals of the week in advance

By setting up a weekly meal plan, you are able to follow a healthy diet with greater ease. Invest some time when you are not busy writing a written meal plan and prepare the corresponding grocery list for each week.

Calculate how much time you have weekly or evening to prepare meals. This can affect the choice of dishes or foods to buy at the supermarket.

Make a schedule for evenings when you are particularly busy; for example, when you decide to go to the gym after work or have a very long meeting that holds you back at work. Try to plan quick meals in advance, that don't require cooking times or that are in any case shortened, for these evenings when you have a lot to do.

Stock up in the kitchen

A well-stocked kitchen is essential to get quick and healthy meals. The less time you waste going to and from the supermarket or looking for ingredients, the better.

Make a full shopping list and go to the store when you're not hungry. Studies have found that this makes it easier to stick to the shopping list and less temptation to buy unhealthy foods and snacks, leaving them on the shelves rather than putting them in the cart.

Always have fruit and vegetables on hand. Whether fresh, frozen or canned, they are all good. Also consider taking ready-made, washed foods, such as lettuce or packaged broccoli buds, to reduce preparation time.

It is also useful to always keep basic products in the kitchen to prepare quick meals. Consider always having on hand canned beans, whole grains (rice or whole grain pasta, quinoa), dressing, sauces, nuts or nut butter. Also, don't rule out the possibility of buying pre-cooked cereals, such as brown rice or quinoa.

Among the quick-to-prepare protein foods are frozen ones (such as chicken or fish), fresh and precooked proteins (such as grilled or sliced chicken strips), canned tuna or chicken. They are all perfect solutions to always have available.

Chapter 25 - Yoga and Intermittent Fasting

Most women over 50 that successfully follow an intermittent fasting protocol decide to include a few yoga training sessions during the week to improve their self awareness and lose more weight at the same time. In this chapter we are going to discuss the basics of this practice and how it can be a good tool to boost your weight loss journey.

The practice of yoga is recognized for its effectiveness in fighting stress and relaxing the mind. However, the more dynamic positions help you burn fat and lose weight. Although the exercises in this discipline do not allow you to burn off calories as effectively as aerobic training, intense sessions and asanas that focus on building muscle strength can be of great help. To begin, choose a type of yoga aimed at strengthening the body and integrate it into your training program. Then, also pay attention to the mental predisposition typically associated with this discipline. Since yoga is effective in encouraging women to live in the present and be aware of their body, it can help limit binges. Although it is healthy and effective in facilitating weight loss, you should never rely solely and exclusively on yoga to lose weight. To shed the extra pounds, it is also necessary to focus on following a healthy intermittent fasting protocol.

Hybrid yoga classes

Yoga alone doesn't burn a lot of calories. Instead, hybrid classes often combine it with aerobic exercise. These variations can promote greater calorie expenditure, helping to burn more calories and perhaps lose weight with the help of yoga.

For instance "koga classes" combine yoga and kickboxing. Since this sport is dynamic and speeds up your heart rate, it can help you burn more calories than yoga alone.

Yoga classes that combine dance and cardiovascular exercises, such as Yoga Booty Ballet, encourage the execution of dynamic movements. If you can find such a class, you may be more likely to lose weight with yoga.

Find out about courses taught in gyms or sports centers in your city. See if you can find one that fits your interests and combines yoga with more vigorous training programs.

Power yoga

It is a form of yoga that requires the performance of demanding athletic poses. It focuses on the muscle groups that need to be used for activities such as cycling, running and weight lifting. If you do power yoga two or three times a week, you will be able to have greater strength and endurance when doing aerobic activities. This will help you burn off more calories both when you engage in other types of workouts and when you move throughout the day.

Acro-yoga

It is a type of yoga combined with acrobatics. It is more intense than other disciplines, as it involves the execution of more complex movements. By helping to burn more calories than traditional yoga, it can be effective in losing weight.

Look for a studio in your city that offers acro-yoga classes. In any case, proceed with caution if you are a beginner. Exercises in this discipline can be quite challenging. If you've never practiced yoga before, you risk getting hurt. In this case it is recommended to start with a beginner course and then gradually move on to acro-yoga.

Hot yoga

This variant can help you lose weight quickly. Hot yoga is generally practiced in a room heated to a temperature of 40° C, with a high level of humidity. While it is useful for shedding excess fluids, there is some controversy as to its actual effectiveness in losing weight over the long term.

Hot yoga sessions are long, lasting around 90 minutes. The longer the duration, the more calories you will burn and consequently the more kilos you will lose.

Hot yoga classes are challenging. Generally, you have to repeat the execution of 26 poses twice. Each pose should be held for 20 seconds the first time and 10 the second.

Look for a hot yoga class in your city and find out how much it costs to see if it's affordable. Practicing it regularly could help you lose weight over time if combined with an intermittent fasting protocol.

The ideal length of the session

Since asanas often involve slow movements, weight loss tends to be less effective. Of course, a 20-minute aerobic workout is much more effective for burning calories than a yoga session of the same length. Consequently, if you want yoga to play a strategic role in your weight loss program, it is essential to practice yoga for 90 minutes at a time. It takes longer sessions to burn more calories and reach your goals.

You should also opt for a more dynamic yoga variant. Look for a course that allows you to perform continuous and steady movements, in order to induce you to maintain a certain rhythm during the session.

You can find yoga classes online or sign up for a class organized by a studio in your city.

Develop muscles through specific poses

Although yoga cannot replace aerobics (it can only complement cardiovascular workouts), it is effective for having a stronger and more toned physique. Developing the muscles and core allows you to strengthen the body. This can help you gain greater endurance, helping you to perform aerobic exercises. In this way the body will be able to sustain longer cardiovascular workouts.

The downward facing dog position helps build muscle mass. This pose is a good starting point for performing similar poses. Rise from the position with your feet together and bend forward at the hips. Proceed until your fingers or palms touch your feet.

Bend your knees and place your palms on the mat, calculating an opening equal to shoulder distance. Then, step back slightly with your feet and push your tailbone towards the ceiling.

Yoga poses at the end of a workout

When you finish exercising, you can perform a quick series of yoga poses. You will thus add targeted exercises to strengthen muscles and enhance cardiovascular training. Choose a set of four or five poses that suit your needs and perform them in a certain order at the end of the workout.

You could start with the mountain position. In a standing position, bring your feet together and stretch your arms over your head. Inhale and exhale as you extend your arms. Starting from the mountain position, lower your arms and bend towards the floor, resting your palms or fingers in front of your feet. Exhale as you lean forward. Tilt your head down and stretch your calves upward.

Look straight ahead, lift your torso and keep your back straight. Push your hips back and switch to the Downward Dog Pose. Then, repeat the circuit.

If you are a beginner, proceed gradually. Yoga is not easy and can put tension on various muscle groups. Certain positions are not recommended for beginners. If you've never practiced this discipline before, it's best to start by signing up for a course. A qualified instructor can help you determine your physical fitness level, giving you advice and opinions on the most suitable positions for your needs.

Greater awareness when you eat

Yoga promotes a greater sense of psychophysical self-awareness. Since it helps to make more careful choices in food, it allows you to consciously determine perceptions such as a sense of satiety and contentment. When you eat, remember to be present in the moment and commit to implementing conscious eating habits.

To get started, make mealtimes a priority. Put your cell phone away and turn off the television. Make equipment (even when you eat alone) to be able to concentrate only on food.

Eat slowly. You need to make sure you savor every bite, welcoming all the sensory factors associated with tasting food with pleasure. Try to chew, pay attention to the taste and texture of what you ingest. Try eating smaller bites and pause between bites to reflect on the present.

Think about the food you eat. Learn to be aware of where it comes from. Who grew the vegetables on your plate? Think about the farms where the animal products come from. Try to think of food in terms of sustenance and nutrition rather than ease or pleasure.

Become more aware of your body

Yoga also teaches you to become more physically aware. This can help you more consciously manage the desire to eat and the choice of foods you need to feel satisfied.

Many dieters struggle to control their body or eating habits. However, according to the teachings of yoga, it is the body that should control you. Yoga classes encourage you to listen to your body and its needs.

When you start practicing yoga regularly, you will realize that you are more aware of what you want and what you need day after day. You will start eating when you are hungry rather than when you feel bored, as you will learn to pay attention to the signals your body sends you. You will also choose healthier foods, because your desire will be to nourish the body rather than research factors such as taste or pleasure.

Before eating, stop and think: "Why am I eating? Am I hungry?". If you eat for other reasons, such as stress, try to find another way to deal with the problem. Eat only when your intermittent fasting protocol allows you to.

Conclusion

We would like to thank you for making it to the end of this intermittent fasting guide. We have done our best to ensure that every information contained is useful and helps you in your journey towards a healthier you.

We know how frustrating it could be to start an intermittent fasting protocol and feeling discouraged by the fact that results do not appear immediately. As we repeated throughout this entire guide, the goal of intermittent fasting is to create a healthy lifestyle that can support you over the years, not just give you a rapid weight loss that is unsustainable over the long run.

By following the intermittent fasting protocols and strategies shared in this book, you will certainly burn fat, lose weight and feel much better. However, as we do not know you in person, our final recommendation can only be the following one.

Before starting an intermittent fasting protocol talk to your doctor and find out whether intermittent fasting could be a good idea for you or not. Remember, never sacrifice your health to fit into that new skirt you just got.

Be healthy and your weight will adapt.

To your success!

Nancy Johnson